KETO AFTER 50 WEIGHT-LOSS PLAN

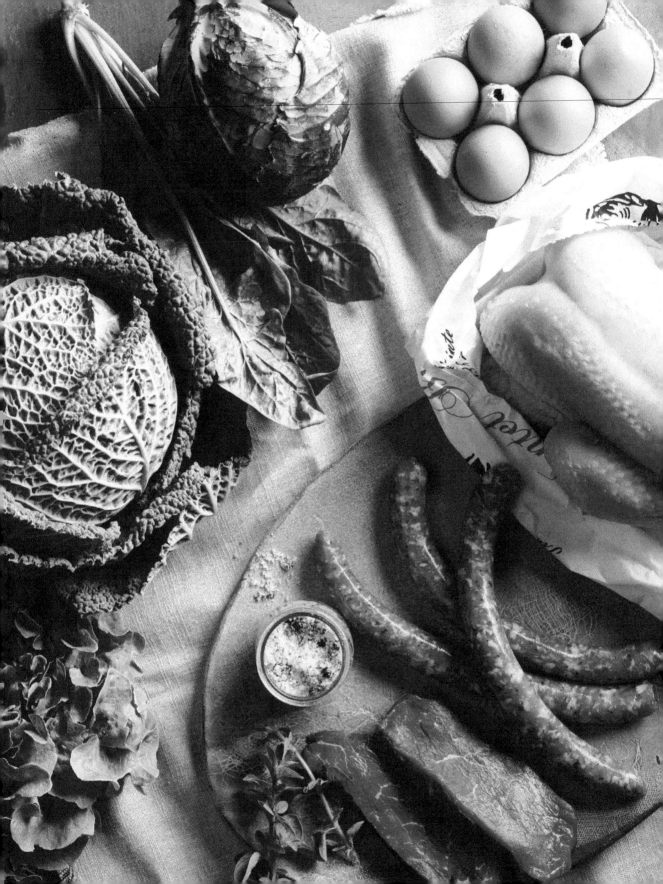

KETO AFTER 50

WEIGHT-LOSS PLAN

28-DAY KETOGENIC DIET PLAN
for a Slimmer, Healthier You

Molly Devine, RD

ROCKRIDGE PRESS

Copyright © 2022 by Rockridge Press

All rights reserved. No part of this publication may be reproduced, stored in a retrieval system, or transmitted in any form or by any means, electronic, mechanical, photocopying, recording, scanning, or otherwise without the prior written permission of the Publisher. Requests to the Publisher for permission should be addressed to the Permissions Department, Rockridge Press, 1955 Broadway, Suite 400, Oakland, CA 94612.

First Rockridge Press trade paperback edition 2022

Rockridge Press and the Rockridge Press logo are trademarks or registered trademarks of Callisto Media Inc. and/or its affiliates in the United States and other countries and may not be used without written permission.

For general information on our other products and services, please contact our Customer Care Department within the United States at (866) 744-2665, or outside the United States at (510) 253-0500.

Paperback ISBN: 978-1-63878-864-5
eBook ISBN: 978-1-63878-530-9

Manufactured in the United States of America

Interior and Cover Designer: Chiaka John
Art Producer: Melissa Malinowsky
Editor: Marjorie DeWitt
Production Editor: Matthew Burnett
Production Manager: Martin Worthington

Photography © 2022 Marija Vidal, food styling by Elisabet der Nederlanden; © Darren Muir, cover; © Alicia Cho, p. xii; Illustrations © Drew Bardana, pp. 160, 161, 162, 163; iStock, pp. x, 48

Author photograph courtesy of Hema Salama Photography

10 9 8 7 6 5 4 3 2 1 0

*For my parents,
whose constant
support means
the world to me*

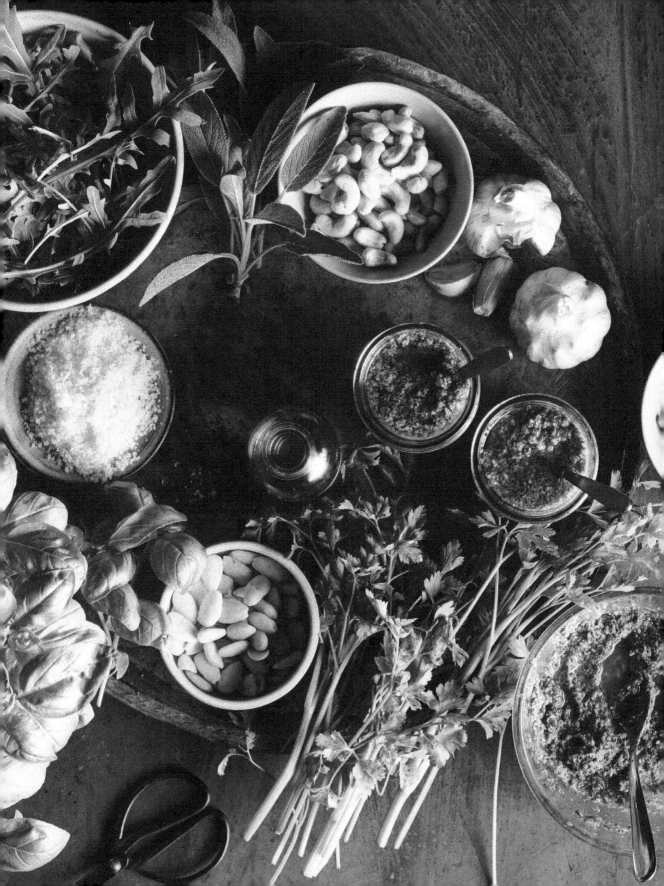

CONTENTS

INTRODUCTION

Losing weight at any age is difficult, but it can feel even more so the older we get. Many of my clients come to me defeated and feeling that weight loss after the age of 50 is nearly impossible. This is understandable, as there is so much conflicting information out there, too many unsustainable fad diets that only result in a feeling of failure, and a belief that part of the natural aging process includes resigning yourself to weight gain and the health implications that can come with that. I am here to help you understand that although weight loss may be more challenging than it was in your younger years, for a variety of reasons, it is far from impossible and only needs to be addressed from a lifestyle perspective rather than a quick-fix diet perspective. Healthy weight loss after 50 *can* be achieved and a well-balanced ketogenic diet can help you realize this goal.

As a registered dietitian specializing in integrative and functional nutrition, I help my clients understand that food is our best medicine and that properly fueling our bodies is the cornerstone to healthy weight maintenance and optimal long-term health. By implementing a well-formulated and nutrient-dense ketogenic diet high in quality healthy fats and low in carbohydrates, my clients are able to feel satiated, reduce cravings, feel more energized for physical activity, and gradually realize their weight-loss goals.

The ketogenic diet has gained popularity in recent years with, often-times, misguided claims of drastic weight loss in a short period of time. This is simply not the reality for any sustainable or healthy weight-loss plan, but when ketogenic lifestyle practices are properly put into place, they can be effective tools to help anyone achieve improved health, body composition, and gradual weight loss that can be maintained long-term.

Setting yourself up for success with realistic expectations is key. In this book, I will help you understand how to create a balanced, varied, and enjoyable ketogenic nutrition plan tailored to meet your goals of healthy weight loss and maintenance over time. I will also help you understand the importance of meal timing, regular body movement, and portion control to allow for progress. Food should taste good, and I want you to enjoy this lifestyle. The recipes in this book will appeal to the novice cook in their simplicity and to the seasoned chef with their abundance of deep flavor and palatability. The 28-day meal plan and 75 easy keto recipes will make following this lifestyle simple and straightforward and give you all the tools you need to kick-start your journey to better health and healthy weight loss.

I hope you come to enjoy the ketogenic lifestyle as much as I do and that you find your improved health and weight-loss progress inspirational for your continued long-term success. Now, let's dive in!

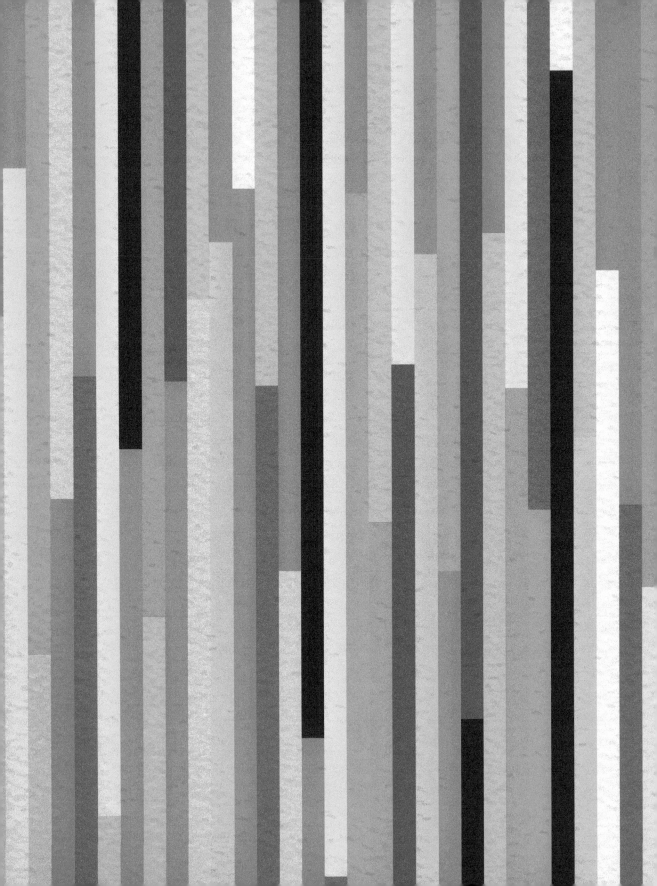

PART ONE

GETTING A NEW START WITH KETO

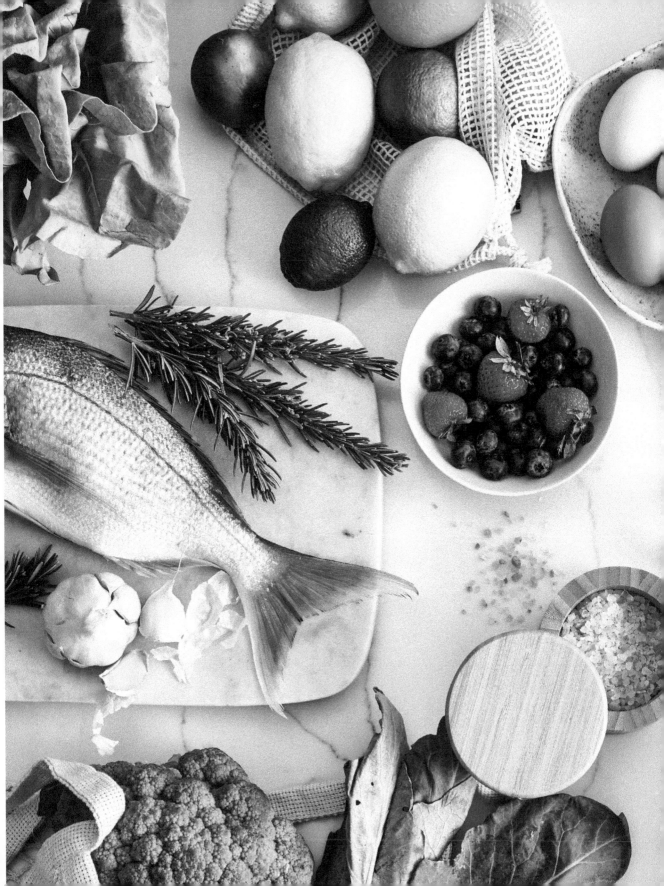

1

WEIGHT LOSS AND THE KETO DIET AFTER 50

Making lifestyle changes is hard work at any age, but with the proper guidance and plan, change doesn't have to feel insurmountable and can even be sustainable lifelong. In this chapter, I will help you understand the many health benefits of going keto after 50 as well as how best to formulate this way of eating to accomplish your weight-loss goals. You can do this, and I'm here to support you.

WHY GO KETO NOW?

The standard American diet, appropriately also referred to as SAD, is the name given to the typical diet followed by most Americans—high in refined carbohydrates, sugars, and processed foods—and is one of the leading causes of chronic disease and obesity in the United States. In a time of busy on-the-go schedules, it is understandable why this has become the norm for so many Americans, but especially as we age, this way of eating promotes constant insulin secretion, making weight gain inevitable. Over time, the complications associated with carrying excess weight, such as joint pain, elevated blood pressure, diabetes, and cardio-vascular disease, begin to emerge.

After 50, you may find that maintaining a healthy weight is becoming more difficult. You may have tried to lose weight in the past but felt frustrated either by the lack of progress or an inability to keep the weight off. Simply put, short-term "diets" don't work. Not only are they often excessively restrictive, leading to regular hunger and a sense of deprivation, but they are also not sustainable and, inevitably, lead to gaining the weight back. As humans, we are impatient and desire immediate results, which often leads people to try the newest fad in an effort to lose weight fast. Weight loss is not a race, but rather a paced event that requires adequate preparation, training, and endurance. A properly formulated and "clean" ketogenic diet allows for progress without excessive calorie restriction while improving other health factors, such as blood sugar control, decreased inflammation and risk for chronic disease, and improved mental clarity and mood.

Many people confuse a ketogenic diet with simply being "low carb," but it is more complex than that. The majority of energy, or calories, consumed on a ketogenic diet comes from dietary fat, only a moderate amount from protein, and a very low amount from carbohydrates. This eliminates completely the refined carbohydrates, sugars, and processed foods that are so prevalent in the SAD, resulting in less circulating insulin and fat storage, reduced inflammation, and more weight loss.

This chapter addresses the ketogenic diet and weight loss in the context of the metabolic needs of anyone over age 50. However, as with any dietary intervention, it is best to check with your doctor or registered dietitian to make sure this lifestyle and way of eating aligns with your specific nutritional and health needs.

HOW DOES KETOSIS WORK?

THE STANDARD AMERICAN DIET: HIGH-CARB

Eat a high carb diet	Blood sugar/ glucose levels rise	Pancreas releases insulin

Insulin shuttles glucose into cells	Burst of energy	Blood sugar crashes leading to cravings, hunger, lethargy

THE KETOGENIC DIET: LOW-CARB

 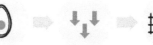

Follow a low-carb, Keto diet	Blood sugar/ glucose levels stabilize and fall over time	Between meals, fat cells release stored fatty acids to convert them to fuel

Fatty acids travel to the liver to be converted into ketones	Ketones travel to cells in the body and brain to be used as energy. Muscle cells use glucose for energy and aren't broken down	Blood sugar and insulin levels are low and stable. Fat is burned/ muscle is spared

THE BENEFITS BEYOND WEIGHT LOSS

Emerging research shows the many benefits of a ketogenic diet for health outcomes and management of many chronic diseases. Specific to the health concerns of those over 50, a well-formulated ketogenic diet can help with:

Blood sugar control. Studies show that by reducing carbohydrate consumption, blood sugar and insulin fluctuations can be reduced as well. By improving insulin control and reversing insulin resistance, improvements in the associated metabolic disorders, such as type 2 diabetes, can be realized.

Long-term cardiac health. For decades, dietary fat, and particularly saturated animal fat, has been labeled the main cause of heart disease, as well as the reason for body fat. However, we are now learning this is not the entire picture. A combination of refined and processed carbohydrates and sugars, as well as high consumption of dietary fats is now known to elevate triglycerides (fat molecules in the blood) and increase the concentration of small particle–size LDL cholesterol. By eating a balanced diet that includes "healthy" fats and limited carbohydrates, it is possible to improve the "good" HDL cholesterol and lower the "bad" LDL cholesterol, which, ultimately, can lower the risk of cardiac disease.

Neurological function. When the body is in ketosis, ketones are used as fuel for the brain, which is a more efficient source of fuel than glucose. This leads to a higher level of alertness and a feeling of being mentally energized throughout the day. For these reasons, the ketogenic diet is being studied for its potential impact on other neurological diseases, including Alzheimer's and Parkinson's diseases.

Reduced joint inflammation (arthritis). Another well-studied benefit of a ketogenic diet is the production of high levels of anti-inflammatory adenosine during metabolism, which is greatly increased in the metabolic state of ketosis. Although many nutrition interventions can bring benefits from the foods they include, a ketogenic diet has the added powerful health benefit of transitioning the body into a new metabolic state that is inherently anti-inflammatory.

Even beyond being a nutrition intervention for the chronic conditions listed here, the ketogenic diet helps improve quality of life in numerous other ways, such as improved sleep due to better blood sugar regulation, hormonal balance due to a reduction in insulin surges, and a decrease in depressive thoughts and enhanced mood due to enhanced brain health and stable energy levels.

HOW WEIGHT LOSS WORKS AFTER 50

To fully understand how the ketogenic diet can contribute to achieving your weight-loss goals, it is important to understand how some changes in our bodies after the age of 50 might impede progress. Understanding these changes, but, more important, their solutions for management, will help you achieve your weight-loss goals.

Slower Metabolism

Although as we age, we do experience a slight decline in basal metabolic rate (BMR), or the baseline calories our bodies burn on a daily basis (not factoring in exercise or activities of daily living), emerging research is showing that this decline is not as sharp as we once thought. The main factors for decreasing metabolism as we age are a more sedentary life-style, lower muscle mass (muscle burns more calories than fat does), and for some, an intake of less nutrient-dense foods. Additionally, those with a history of yo-yo or restrictive dieting in their younger years will experience a decreased metabolic rate over time.

> *The Solution: Stick to eating well-balanced ketogenic meals instead of frequent "empty-calorie" snacks. The satiating healthy fats that are the backbone of a well-balanced ketogenic diet provide adequate calories to keep metabolic function optimal while decreasing hunger and cravings for junk foods.*

Loss of Muscle Mass

Our body composition changes as we age. Lean muscle mass decreases and fat mass and visceral fat around the abdomen increase. These changes not only increase the risk for cardiovascular disease (CVD), high blood pressure, and type 2 diabetes, but also contribute to poor bone health and a reduced metabolism.

> *The Solution: Include regular strength-training or weight-bearing activity as well as adequate quality protein intake to promote weight loss that spares your muscles.*

Hormonal Changes

For many women, hormonal shifts during perimenopause, menopause, and post-menopause can cause insulin levels to shift, making fat storage, specifically in the midsection, more prevalent. Similarly, the negative effect these hormonal changes can have on sleep and stress levels can hinder metabolic function and increase hunger.

The Solution: The high healthy fat/very low carbohydrate makeup of a ketogenic diet reduces levels of circulating insulin and helps eliminate the drastic spikes in insulin that result from a high-sugar/high-carbohydrate standard American diet (SAD), which assists in balancing hormone levels and promoting fat burn rather than fat storage.

Less-Active Lifestyle

Many people find themselves at the height of their careers as they enter their 50s and the demands of office life, travel, and other factors lead to a more sedentary lifestyle than in previous decades. Not only does this cause weight gain from an imbalance of caloric burn versus caloric intake, but often the stress of work-life balance can cause many individuals to turn to emotional or stress eating, increasing overall intake to unhealthy levels.

The Solution: Break the cycle of limited movement and poor eating habits by being more mindful of balanced meal intake and regular movement through the meal plans and simple exercises outlined in the following chapters. These initiatives will result in improvements not only in body composition and weight loss, but mood and energy levels as well. The more we move, the better we feel, which means wanting to move more.

CALCULATING YOUR RATIO

Macronutrients, or *macros* for short, are the building blocks of our diet: proteins, fats, and carbohydrates. To achieve a state of metabolic ketosis, you want the majority of calories in your diet to be derived from fat, a moderate amount from protein, and a bare minimum from carbohydrates. This combination will help you stay fuller longer, prevent cravings and hunger between meals, and allow for weight loss through portion control and reduced overall consumption.

Long-term success for anyone on a ketogenic diet depends on modification and individualization. However, I always start my clients on a basic macronutrient ratio plan to induce ketosis as quickly as possible, kick carb cravings, and start to see improvements in body composition. Specifically for people over 50, I recommend following a 70-20-10 ratio of fat-protein-total carbohydrate. This ratio is high enough in fat to help curb cravings and create satiety, adequate in protein for those over 50 who have increased needs with age, but not so high to prevent ketosis, and low enough in carbs to allow for immediate results. For someone on a 1,200- to 1,400-calorie-per-day meal plan, to allow for weight loss (such as the meal plans in chapter 3), this translates into 90 to 110 grams of fat daily, 60 to 70 grams of protein daily, and under 40 grams of total carbohydrates daily.

HOW THE KETOGENIC DIET HELPS

This section reviews the principles of a ketogenic diet for weight loss and helps you understand the breakdown of the 70-20-10 macronutrient ratio explained in the sidebar on page 7 and how to get the most out of each of these groups to meet your nutrient needs as someone over 50.

Low Carb

Because only 10 percent or less of your daily calories will come from carbohydrates and they are the main macronutrient in non-starchy veggies and low-sugar fruits, these foods should be the backbone of your daily carbohydrate consumption.

> **Considerations after 50:** *The overwhelming majority of carbohydrates in your diet should come from whole foods such as non-starchy vegetables and low-sugar fruits like berries, which not only contain fiber but also a host of micronutrients, such as vitamins and minerals, essential to hormone balance and blood pressure regulation as we age. For this reason, I have my clients focus on total carbs over "net carbs" (total carb grams minus fiber grams), the latter of which carry little nutritional value and contain a lot of gut-disrupting sweeteners and chemical additives.*

High Fat

The majority of your daily calories, about 70 percent, will come from quality fat sources.

> **Considerations after 50:** *Fat is the main source of energy in any ketogenic diet, but, as we age, the type of fat is even more important to maintain heart health and decrease inflammation. Saturated fats from animal sources are fine to include in moderation, but the majority of fats should come from unsaturated, heart-healthy fats, such as those found in avocado, fatty fish, olive oil, nuts, and seeds.*

Moderate Protein

One of the biggest differences between a ketogenic diet and a simple low-carb/high-protein diet is the moderation of protein. This moderation is needed because our bodies will turn excess protein (and in small amounts, excess fat) into glucose for use as fuel *before* producing ketones. This process is called *gluconeogenesis* and is a normal daily process, even for those on a ketogenic diet, because glucose is essential for a number of bodily functions. Most people overconsume protein thinking that it only goes to their muscles. In fact, most people cannot absorb more than 25 to 35 grams of protein per meal, which amounts to only 4 to 6 ounces of meat or fish.

> **Considerations after 50:** *Many older adults suffer from high blood pressure (hypertension), which can be exacerbated by an excessively high-sodium diet. Avoiding large quantities of highly processed meats, such as hot dogs, deli meats, and bacon, and focusing on quality free-range and grass-fed poultry, meats, and eggs, as well as wild-caught seafood, helps keep sodium levels in check and reduces the risk for hypertension.*

Lots of Micronutrients

Vitamins and minerals, or micronutrients, are important to overall health, especially as we age. Ensuring ample amounts of colorful non-starchy vegetables and low-sugar fruits in your meals will help you hit an optimal level of nutrition every day.

> **Considerations after 50:** *Many "dirty keto" diets rely heavily on processed and packaged keto products instead of colorful plants as the main source of carbohydrates. These diets lack the essential fiber, vitamins, and minerals integral for bone, skin, metabolic, and digestive health, especially as we age.*

ALL ABOUT KETOSIS

When you stop supplying your body with glucose from carbohydrates, it will need to look for a new fuel source for energy and cell function. Not all cells can use pure fatty acids for fuel, and most importantly, the brain cannot use them at all. Ketosis is the body's natural metabolic process of converting these fatty acids into usable currency for energy: a ketone. Fatty acids travel to the liver, where they are converted into ketones and sent throughout the body for use as energy. Ketones are like the rocket fuel of gas; they are extremely efficient, provide long-term energy, and improve function.

Achieving ketosis is different for everyone and varies based on previous carbohydrate intake, body composition, insulin resistance, and fitness level. Following the meal plans outlined in chapter 3 should allow your body to enter ketosis within 3 to 5 days, but achieving and maintaining a high level of ketosis is not vital for weight loss on a ketogenic diet. The increased fats will provide satiety. And when your brain is fueled by ketones (from the conversion of fatty acids as described previously), not glucose, it stops craving or looking for a steady stream of carbohydrate and sugar-dense foods. Not only do these factors help make avoiding carb-dense foods easier, but hunger is also reduced as your body adapts to utilizing stored energy (from body fat) for fuel between meals, making portion control manageable and the need for frequent meals and snacks obsolete. Reduced intake is the key to weight loss on a ketogenic diet, not necessarily the level of ketones in your blood or urine. For this reason, testing these levels is not necessary as long as you see progress with your weight-loss goals.

WHAT TO EAT ON THE KETO DIET

As with any healthy nutrition plan, it is important to emphasize quality and balance in the foods included, as well as to avoid those that can cause damage or prevent progress with health goals. "Dirty keto" is the name given by industry professionals to the imbalanced, often highly processed, and potentially very unhealthy versions of this otherwise promising way of eating. A well-formulated ketogenic diet for overall health and weight loss does not mean just taking the bun off your fast-food hamburger, substituting artificial sweetener in your favorite dessert recipe, or avoiding all vegetables for fear of breaking macro ratios. Rather, a "clean keto" meal plan includes a wide variety of foods, including colorful vegetables, healthy protein sources, and plant-based unsaturated heart-healthy fats while keeping fats from saturated sources, such as dairy and high-fat meats, in moderation. Following these tips for each macronutrient will help keep your plan easy to follow and help you see the progress you desire.

Fat sources: High fat doesn't mean unlimited bacon, butter, cream, and steak. The most beneficial and sustainable ketogenic diet is rich in heart-healthy unsaturated fats from plant and marine sources such as avocado, fatty fish, nuts, olive oil, and seeds.

Protein sources: The best sources of quality animal proteins are fatty fish such as sardines, salmon, mackerel, and anchovies, free-range eggs high in omega-3 fatty acids, free-range poultry, and grass-fed meats, which are all high in heart-healthy fats. Seeds and nuts are great sources of plant-based proteins and are also loaded with heart-healthy omega-3 fatty acids. Remember, on a ketogenic diet, we moderate how much protein is consumed, so a little can go a long way.

Carbohydrate sources: I emphasize the importance of plant-based carbohydrates, such as non-starchy vegetables and low-sugar fruits, rather than processed keto-friendly packaged food products. The former are chock-full of micronutrients (vitamins and minerals), which are essential for cell function, digestion, metabolism, and overall health to fuel workouts and performance. The latter tend to be mostly "filler fibers" that the body cannot process well, chemicals and additives such as artificial sweeteners and dyes, and inflammatory fats. For this reason, I don't look at "net carbs," but rather total carbs as the best number to watch. The carbohydrates in your diet should come primarily from whole foods such as dark leafy greens, colorful fruits and veggies such as berries and bell peppers, and fibers found in nuts and seeds for maximum health benefit.

FOODS TO EAT AND AVOID ON KETO

	FOODS TO EAT REGULARLY	FOODS TO EAT OCCASIONALLY	FOODS TO AVOID
VEGETABLES	Asparagus; celery; cruciferous vegetables (e.g., broccoli, Brussels sprouts, cauliflower); eggplant; fennel; garlic; green beans; leafy greens (e.g., arugula, kale, radicchio lettuces, spinach); mushrooms; onions; pickles; radish; summer squash (zucchini and yellow squash)	Bell peppers (¼-cup serving); carrots (¼-cup serving); pumpkin and other winter squash (½-cup serving); tomatoes (¼-cup serving)	Corn; peas; potatoes; yams
FISH AND SEAFOOD	All, with an emphasis on high-fat wild-caught fish, such as anchovies, salmon, sardines, and tuna canned in olive oil		
MEATS AND PROTEINS	Free-range eggs; free-range poultry; grass-fed beef and lamb; pasture-raised pork	Nitrate-free cured meats like all-beef hot dogs, bacon, deli meat, salami, etc.	Nitrate-containing processed meats like bacon, deli meats, and sausage containing sugar or other fillers
DAIRY AND CHEESE	Full-fat cheese (limit to 1 ounce per meal); full-fat cream cheese (limit to 1 ounce per meal); grass-fed butter (limit to 2 tablespoons per meal); heavy (whipping) cream (limit to 2 tablespoons per meal); sour cream (limit to 2 tablespoons per meal)	Full-fat cottage cheese (⅓-cup serving); whole milk Greek or Icelandic yogurt (½-cup serving)	Milk; processed cheeses such as low-fat or part-skim cheese and cream cheese; sweetened yogurt

	FOODS TO EAT REGULARLY	FOODS TO EAT OCCASIONALLY	FOODS TO AVOID
GRAINS AND LEGUMES			All, except peanuts
FRUITS	Avocados, berries (e.g., blackberries, blueberries, raspberries, strawberries); lemons; limes	Dark cherries (limit to 5 per serving); oranges and clementines (½ orange or 1 small clementine)	Higher-sugar fruits (e.g., apples, melon, peaches, pears, plums)
NUTS, SEEDS, AND FLOURS	All tree nuts and nut butters (e.g., almonds, Brazil nuts, cashews, coconuts, filberts/hazelnuts, macadamia nuts, pecans, pine nuts, walnuts); chia, flax and hemp seeds; pumpkin seeds; sesame seeds and tahini (sesame seed paste)	Almond flour; coconut flour	Chickpea flour, rice flour, white flour, whole wheat flour
FATS AND OILS	Avocado oil; avocado or olive oil–based mayonnaise; coconut oil and full-fat unsweetened coconut milk; MCT oil; olive oil; olives		Processed vegetable oils (e.g., canola, corn, soybean)
SWEETENERS, SPICES, AND SEASONINGS	Apple cider and red wine vinegars; herbs (fresh or dried) such as basil, mint, parsley, rosemary, etc.; unsweetened spices and seasonings such as black pepper, chili powder, cinnamon, red pepper flakes, salt; stone-ground mustard; unsweetened hot sauce; vanilla extract; Worcestershire sauce	Balsamic vinegar (1 tablespoon per serving); monk fruit; stevia; sugar alcohols (erythritol, sorbitol)	Artificial sweeteners (Splenda, Sweet'N Low); barbecue sauce; ketchup; seasoning blends that include sugar (e.g., cinnamon sugar blend); sugar of any kind (agave, brown sugar, cane sugar, corn syrup, honey, maple syrup)

FAQ AND TROUBLESHOOTING

Even with the best of intentions and a well-formulated plan, changing the way you eat can feel overwhelming at first, and that is to be expected. This section covers the common mistakes I often see arise when my clients start keto for the first time.

Stay hydrated! The quick dumping of stored water as the body breaks down stored glycogen within the first few days of starting a ketogenic diet can lead to dehydration from a loss of electrolytes along with the water. As a general rule, I suggest drinking water equivalent to half your body weight in ounces daily. So, if you weigh 200 pounds, aim for about 100 ounces of water a day. This can come in the form of unsweetened teas, seltzers, or fruit-infused waters along with plain old tap water. If properly hydrated, electrolyte replacement is not usually necessary, but if you are feeling low energy, achy, and light-headed, you may want to include an electrolyte replacement (see page 28).

Attack carb or sugar cravings with fat. If you have a craving for something carb heavy or find yourself hungry between meals, attack it with a fatty snack, such as those listed in chapter 8, or a simple high-fat food like half an avocado with a sprinkle of salt, which has an added electrolyte bonus of potassium in the avocado and sodium in the salt, or celery sticks with peanut butter. You are trying to retrain your cells and brain to look for fat as a primary fuel source rather than glucose from carbs. By giving it fat when a craving for quick energy hits, you reinforce this process and encourage your body to make the transition.

Don't go hungry. Even though we are focusing on portion control for weight loss, the first few days or weeks after starting a ketogenic diet can be tricky and you may find yourself in need of an extra fat serving at meals, such as dressing on a salad, avocado on eggs, or olive oil on sautéed veggies. Cravings will lessen and natural satiety will take over as your body becomes more fat adapted, but in the first week or two, don't worry about those extra fat servings to keep cravings and hunger at bay.

Eat real foods and don't focus on net carbs. The overwhelming majority of carbohydrates in the ideal diet should come from real foods, such as non-starchy vegetables, which contain fiber in addition to a host of vitamins and minerals essential to healthy metabolic function and overall cell function. I recommend avoiding all boxed "keto-friendly" commercial products that tout low "net carbs," such as bars, breads, cereals, cookies, and wraps and, instead, exploring the delicious, real food recipes in the chapters that follow. Your body will feel and function so much better, and many of those processed foods won't even taste good anymore.

Avoid "cheat days," but being social and indulging here and there is okay. You can take your ketogenic lifestyle to the party or restaurant, but I encourage you not to give in to the desire for an all-out "cheat day," which usually spirals out of control quickly and, for many, can be a slippery slope. This digression will also negate any weight-loss progress made. Remember, carbs are just a form of quick energy, so if you overdo it in one meal, include a fasted workout the next morning to burn any remaining glucose and stored glycogen and get back on track with your meal plan.

Keep alcohol in moderation. Although many wines and spirits are low in carbohydrates, the body prioritizes the processing and burning of alcohol over any other energy source, including fat. The liver is also the organ responsible for the conversion of fatty acids to ketones for energy, so if it is busy detoxifying from the alcohol, it won't be effective at making ketones and will halt the ketogenic process. Aside from the metabolic downsides of excessive alcohol consumption, alcohol is dehydrating, inflammatory, and can cause more carb and sugar cravings.

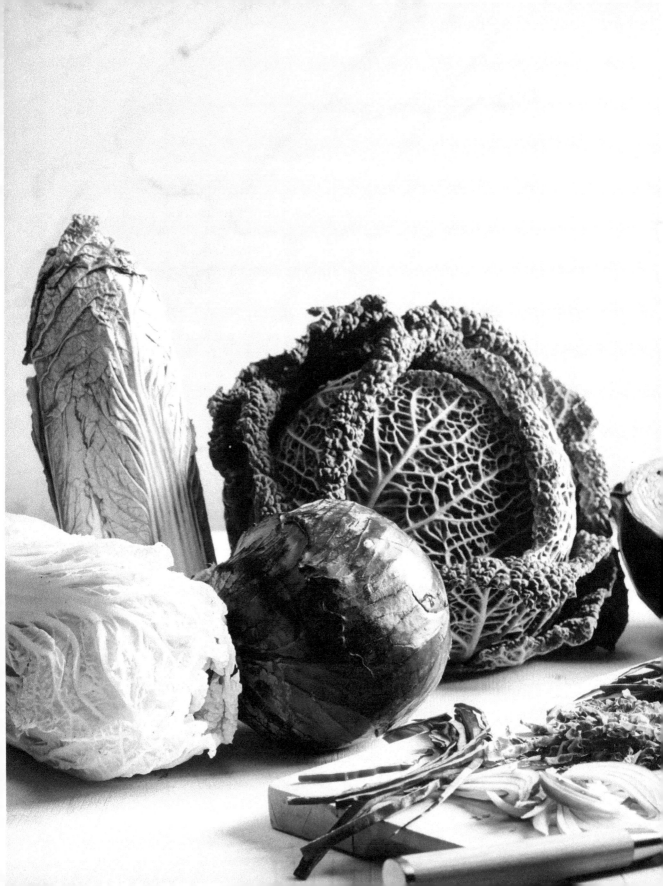

2

PREPARING FOR SUCCESS

The key to any successful weight-loss journey is preparation. Stressful, busy days will happen, but when you have properly stocked your pantry, refrigerator, and freezer with convenient keto-friendly options and planned your meals in advance, such days don't have to derail you. The following chapter will help set you up for success on your ketogenic plan for weight loss.

STOCKING YOUR KETO PANTRY

The recipes in this book are designed to be easy to follow and use minimal ingredients, but there are some basic pantry staples I recommend keeping on hand to make it all flow seamlessly.

Almond flour: This low-carb, grain-free flour is high in protein and fat. Almond flour is great for keto-friendly baked goods and treats and as a thickener in savory recipes.

Arrowroot powder: A thickening agent, like cornstarch, but lower in carbohydrate, arrowroot powder is in some of the sauces and baked goods recipes in this book.

Avocados: Loaded with heart-healthy fats, fiber, and dehydration-preventing potassium, I consider this keto superfood a pantry staple because you should store unripe avocados in a dark place at room temperature. Once they start to ripen, move the avocados to the refrigerator so they last longer before browning.

Baking powder: Not just for sweets and baked goods, you'll use baking powder in some baked egg and cheese dishes to give them volume and optimal texture.

Canned diced tomatoes and no-sugar-added tomato sauce: Although tomatoes do contain natural sugars (carbs), a little goes a long way toward boosting flavor. Canned options are great when fresh tomatoes are not in season.

Canned seafood (tuna, sardines, salmon, anchovies): Heart-healthy fatty fish packed in olive oil is a tasty, convenient, and portable protein option on the go. Topping mixed greens with canned tuna, avocado, and a drizzle of olive oil is my favorite 2-minute no-recipe meal in a pinch.

Oils: Heart-healthy extra-virgin olive oil or avocado oil is best for most cooking and sautéing. Coconut oil is also used for its great flavor, particularly in baked goods.

Spices and dried herbs: These ingredients bring massive flavor. Ones you'll see frequently in this book include cinnamon, cumin, curry powder, garlic powder, Italian seasoning, onion powder, oregano, pumpkin pie spice, and thyme.

Stock or broth (beef, chicken, and vegetable): Keep these on hand in your pantry for homemade soups and stews. Bone stock or broth also makes a great hot beverage to help replenish electrolytes and overcome a "keto flu" (see page 28).

Sugar-free sweeteners: These are always optional, but best used in baked goods and treats. If you are trying to wean your palate off a high-sugar diet, you may find adding some sugar-free sweetener to beverages and yogurt is helpful. I prefer stevia- and monk fruit–based versions such as Swerve. Brands that include sugar alcohols, such as erythritol, can be upsetting to the gut when consumed in high doses.

Unsweetened nut and seed butters: Not only are butters such as almond, cashew, sunflower, and tahini (sesame seed paste) used in many recipes in this book for flavor, but they make a great snack in a pinch.

Vinegars: Keep balsamic vinegar, red wine vinegar, and rice wine vinegar on hand for homemade dressings, marinades, and sauces.

KETO-FRIENDLY ALTERNATIVES

I really stress the importance of "whole foods" for any successful nutrition plan, and so many of the "keto products" out there aren't what I would call whole foods, because they are often high in filler fibers and chemicals that may delay progress. Rather than seek out an exact replica for favorite carb- and sugar-heavy foods, rethink your approach and look for plant-based whole foods to take their place.

BREAD, ROLLS, WRAPS FOR SANDWICHES	Cheese-based wraps such as Folio brand, Everything but the Carb Bread (page 150), lettuce or cabbage leaf wraps
BREAKFAST CEREALS INCLUDING OATMEAL	Chopped nuts atop plain yogurt, N'Oatmeal (page 57)
CHIPS, CRACKERS, AND OTHER CRUNCHY SNACK FOODS	Kale chips, raw veggies such as bell pepper, broccoli, carrots in moderation, celery, and cucumber, nuts, Rosemary and Olive Oil Crackers (page 146)
PASTA, RICE, AND OTHER GRAINS	Riced cauliflower, shirataki "miracle" noodles, thin French green beans, thinly sliced cabbage, zucchini noodles
SAUCES AND DRESSINGS WITH ADDED SUGARS	Aioli sauces or flavored mayonnaise, Creamy Caesar Dressing (page 154), infused olive or avocado oil, no-sugar-added marinara sauce such as Rao's, pesto, soy or tamari sauce, tahini (sesame seed paste), vinegar
SODA AND OTHER SWEETENED BEVERAGES	Herbal teas (hot or iced), no-sugar-added electrolyte beverages such as G2 or Powerade Zero, unsweetened carbonated water such as LaCroix
SWEET TREATS	Almond butter or other nut butters, berries and whipped cream, dark chocolate (85 percent cocoa or higher), desserts or treats in moderation, such as Keto Granola Bites (page 147)

MEAL PLANNING AND PREPPING

One of the best ways to ensure success with this new lifestyle and way of eating is to plan and prep meals ahead. No one makes the best dietary choices when they are overly hungry and the refrigerator is empty. Knowing what is on the menu and having the ingredients and materials you need will keep you on track and help you achieve your weight-loss goals.

Meal Planning

Putting your goals into action starts with a solid plan.

1. **Determine what meals you need.** The meal plans in chapter 3 give you great structure to get started on a ketogenic weight-loss plan, but they should be customized to your needs and lifestyle. For example, if you are fine eating the same breakfast or lunch daily, you may choose to make fewer recipes each week by doubling up on those that really speak to you. You may also need to look at your schedule for the week to see what commitments may make more convenient keto-friendly meals better options on those days.

2. **Start thinking about recipes based on ingredients you have, seasonality, or what's on sale.** Food sticker shock is lost on no one. I get my local grocery store's circular sent to my email inbox weekly and plan my family's meals for the week based on what is on sale. The meal plans that follow provide a guide for jump-starting your weight-loss journey, but you can be flexible on the proteins and veggies included, and choose some recipes over others based on seasonality and availability. For example, feel free to sub pork loin chops for chicken thighs, ground beef or dark meat chicken for ground pork, or tuna for salmon, etc. As you get the hang of this new way of eating, my goal for you is flexibility with ingredients to make them work for you and your lifestyle.

3. **Finalize recipe selections based on maximizing ingredient reuse.** The meal plans in chapter 3 try to make the best use of ingredients to avoid waste, but if you find yourself with extras of a certain perishable ingredient, such as cilantro or arugula, switch up some of the recipes that week to maximize what you have a surplus of.

Meal Prepping

Meal prepping is putting the tires to the road. Not everyone wants or is able to prepare a week's worth of meals in one day. That's okay! Meal prepping can also mean having your ingredients on hand and accessible for later use. The following are my tips for meal prepping for busy weeks:

COOK ONCE, ENJOY MANY TIMES. Repurposing certain components of a dish into a variety of dishes can be a huge timesaver and cut down on frequent cooking. For example, make my Stovetop Chopped Pork Barbecue (page 112) or Curry Roasted Chicken Thighs (page 105) for dinner during the week and repurpose the leftovers atop salads or in lettuce wraps for lunch throughout the week.

PREP AHEAD AND SCALE RECIPES. Picking a day of the week to prep staples, like chopped onions and fresh herbs, and cut veggies, can save significant time getting meals on the table during the week. And, even better, by doing it all at once, you also cut down on cleaning time. Likewise, if you double one or two recipes every week—my Creamy Butternut Soup (page 82) scales especially well—and freeze the leftovers in single-serve portions, over time, you will build up the healthiest array of ready-to-go frozen entrées.

KEEP SAUCES AND DRESSINGS ON HAND. I also love to make sauces, like Versatile Pesto (page 149), and dressings, like Creamy Caesar Dressing (page 154), ahead to be used throughout the week to jazz up simple leftovers, roasted veggies, or a side salad.

CONVENIENT KETO PRODUCTS

I do not advocate filling your diet with commercial "keto" products to attain weight-loss goals. So many of these products have filler ingredients that will delay progress and can even cause weight gain, and many are not, in fact, keto-friendly at all, but I do suggest the following "whole foods" products for convenience and on-the-go meals and snacks.

- Jarred pesto (preferably made with olive oil rather than canola oil)

- Miracle Noodles

- Natural almond butter (unsweetened); Justin's small single-serve packs to keep in the car, or store brand with only almonds and salt as ingredients

- Rao's Marinara, or any bottled marinara sauce with total sugars under 6 grams per serving

- Store-bought hard-boiled eggs

- Store-bought rotisserie chicken

OTHER LIFESTYLE FACTORS FOR WEIGHT LOSS

As much as we'd like to try, you can't outrun a bad diet. For too many years, we have been led to believe in the "calories in–calories out" mentality toward weight loss: If we just exercise enough and eat less, we'll lose weight. Not so. Weight loss and healthy weight maintenance are 80 percent nutrition and 20 percent lifestyle, including factors such as exercise, stress, and sleep. Even if nutrition is on point, a sedentary lifestyle, stressful job, and poor sleep patterns will delay, if not negate, progress. Similarly, exercising an hour a day but not paying attention to your nutrition will not bring any significant or sustainable results. The following sections discuss how to build your complete wheel of health.

Exercise

As discussed in the previous chapter, maintaining an active lifestyle, including regular strength training or weight-bearing exercises, helps offset the natural loss of lean body mass and decline in metabolic rate seen as we age. After age 50, it is more important than ever to have a regular physical activity routine to achieve optimal health and weight for the long-term.

Most people do experience an adjustment phase as they ease into a ketogenic diet, no matter their activity level, so it is so important to be patient with your body and remember that slow and steady wins the race. I am a huge advocate for routine and consistency at first over duration and intensity. In other words, you are better off committing to a light 10-minute walk every day for the first few weeks rather than aiming for 1-hour treadmill sessions on the highest incline. Set realistic expectations, ease into your new routine, and allow your body the time to adjust to your new lifestyle.

CARDIOVASCULAR EXERCISE (CARDIO)

Cardiovascular exercise gets its name from its ability to strengthen the heart and muscles and includes a wide variety of activities like cycling, dancing, rowing, running, swimming, and walking. Some other benefits of cardio include boosting mood through the release of endorphins, improving sleep, reduced stress, and healthy weight management through caloric burn. No matter your fitness level or goals, including some cardio exercise in your routine can improve your overall health and longevity.

During bouts of cardio, the primary fuel source for our bodies is fat. In fact, during periods of rest and daily activities such as light walking, cleaning, and sleeping, fats (both dietary as well as stored) account for 80 to 90 percent of supplied energy. For this reason, while in a state of ketosis through dietary changes or fasting, we are able to supply our bodies easily with the necessary fuel for basic daily function without the need for carbohydrates, making cardiovascular exercise the optimal form of movement on a ketogenic diet geared toward weight loss.

Although cardio does favor fat for fuel, if you are new to a ketogenic diet, it may take time for your body to transition to increased exercise without a steady level of carbohydrates. This is completely normal and, as mentioned previously, you need to ease into this transition. At first, you may not be able to work out for as long or at the same pace as you were previously able to. Don't beat yourself up—listen to your body. Sticking to the plan and routine of low-intensity, short-duration cardio will help your body transition more quickly, usually within one to four weeks.

STRENGTH TRAINING

The natural process of losing lean body mass (muscle) and gaining fat mass as we age can be combated, in part, with a regular strength training or body-resistance workout routine. These activities include using free weights, resistance bands, or weight machines. Not only does strength training help you retain and build lean body mass, but it also helps with bone density and can increase metabolism long-term leading to healthy weight maintenance.

Those new to a ketogenic diet will find that heavy weightlifting or body building routines may be hard to maintain, initially, as you transition away from a carbohydrate-based diet, because glucose is the primary fuel used by muscles for this type of activity. However, those just getting started with strength training or resistance activities should not have a problem engaging in light-weight, low-intensity and short-duration strength training activities despite the lack of excess carbohydrates in their diet.

I will go over in more detail suggested exercises and activities to meet these goals in the Exercises section (see page 158), but as a good place to start, I encourage you to aim for a minimum of five minutes of weight-bearing or body-resistance activity three to five times a week. If you don't have access to weights or bands, perform simple exercises like modified push-ups (using a wall, stairs, or on your knees) or lunges, pull-ups, or squats without weight, or even using soup cans in place of weights for bicep curls.

STRETCHING AND INJURY PREVENTION

Activities like stretching and light yoga may not elevate your heart rate the way cardio and strength training exercises do, but they engage important muscle groups and are vital to elongating muscles, maintaining strength, and preventing injury. I suggest a three- to five-minute light stretch both before and after any exercise. You will find examples in the following chapter, but simple stretching exercises such as touching your toes, or even simple neck and shoulder rolls, will help you gain flexibility and prevent muscle tears.

It is also important to incorporate rest days into your exercise routine as this time allows your muscles to recover, adapt, and grow stronger from the work you've put in. I recommend at least one rest day each week. This can be a day off completely from exercise while keeping your nutrition plan strong, or it can include light walking, stretching, or light yoga, if you prefer.

Sleep

Too many people underestimate the power of a good night's sleep. Not only does quality sleep help us maintain energy levels, mood regulation, and performance, but it also helps with hormone regulation, metabolic function, and keeping hunger at bay. When we are chronically sleep deprived, our ghrelin (also known as the "hunger hormone") levels are elevated, blood sugar is elevated, insulin spikes, and we overeat and go into fat-storage mode. Despite best nutrition and physical activity efforts, weight loss becomes impossible without quality sleep.

To improve sleep hygiene, follow these guidelines:

- Stick to a regular bedtime and waketime routine, regardless of the day. You can't stockpile sleep, so trying to get it all on the weekends or vacation days simply doesn't work and often throws off meal times and other routines.

- Avoid all electronics 30 minutes before bedtime. Aside from the stress that social media and other electronic outlets can bring, the blue light from TVs, cell phones, tablets, and other devices activates neuroreceptors in our brain that prevent us from settling down.

- Aim to have your last meal of the day at least one hour before bedtime to avoid digestive discomfort and shifts in blood sugar that can disrupt sleep.

- Set a goal of six to eight hours of sleep nightly.

Stress

Cortisol is our "fight-or-flight" stress hormone and although it was a life-saving advantage when we were hunting and gathering and running for our lives from a hungry bear, high circulating cortisol levels have become a hinderance to weight loss for many people in an era of constant daily stress. Like poor sleep patterns, high stress levels are often overlooked as a key piece to the puzzle of weight loss and healthy weight maintenance.

In our hectic lives, self-care often gets categorized as a luxury, but I promise you it is imperative to your overall health and weight-loss goals. Whether through physical activity, meditation, reading, journaling, drawing, listening to music, or a relaxing bath, it is important to help your body handle and mitigate everyday stress. For my clients who don't know where to start with stress-relieving practices, I suggest simply closing your eyes for two minutes, taking deep breaths, allowing you to refocus upon opening your eyes. For others, taking a short five-minute walk while listening to your favorite song between meetings works wonders to help decompress.

DEALING WITH KETO FLU

If you've tried keto in the past but had to stop because you felt so horrible in the early days, you likely experienced the "keto flu." Symptoms include nausea, fatigue, headache, and light-headedness and usually start three to four days in and can last anywhere from one to two weeks. This phenomenon is due to the quick dumping of stored water as the body breaks down glycogen stores within the first few days of a very low carbohydrate diet. Although uncomfortable, keto flu is not cause for alarm, and—more important—can be avoided entirely with these tips:

Stay hydrated. As a general rule, I suggest drinking half your body weight in ounces of water each day. So, if you weigh 200 pounds, aim for 100 ounces of water per day, which can come in the form of unsweetened teas, seltzers, or fruit-infused waters.

Keep up with your electrolytes. The main four are calcium, magnesium, potassium, and sodium. And although there are many electrolyte supplement drinks available, many have added sugars, so aim to get your electrolytes from your diet. Avocados are high in potassium and magnesium. Nuts, seeds, and fatty fish, like salmon and tuna packed in oil, are good sources of magnesium. Chicken or beef stock, which are high in sodium, also boost electrolytes. However, if you are on a medically supervised low-sodium diet, consult your doctor before increasing sodium levels.

WHAT TO EXPECT FROM THE PLAN

Changing habits is hard work. Not every day will go smoothly and that is okay. Measuring progress on a scale daily will likely be defeating. You can expect some water weight loss initially from depletion of glycogen stores (see page 14) but this level of weight loss will not and should not be sustained over the long term. I also encourage all my clients to focus on non-scale victories, such as reduced inflammation, reduced cravings, increased energy, and improved mood and mental clarity. As I have mentioned previously, weight loss is not a race, but a journey to be taken in stride. Weight loss also varies for each individual and sometimes a plateau is natural. If you continue to see improvements to other health markers, I encourage you to stay the course and continue to follow your new lifestyle plan. Plateaus are often overcome with consistency and patience but may take up to a month to see continued progress before reaching your healthy goal.

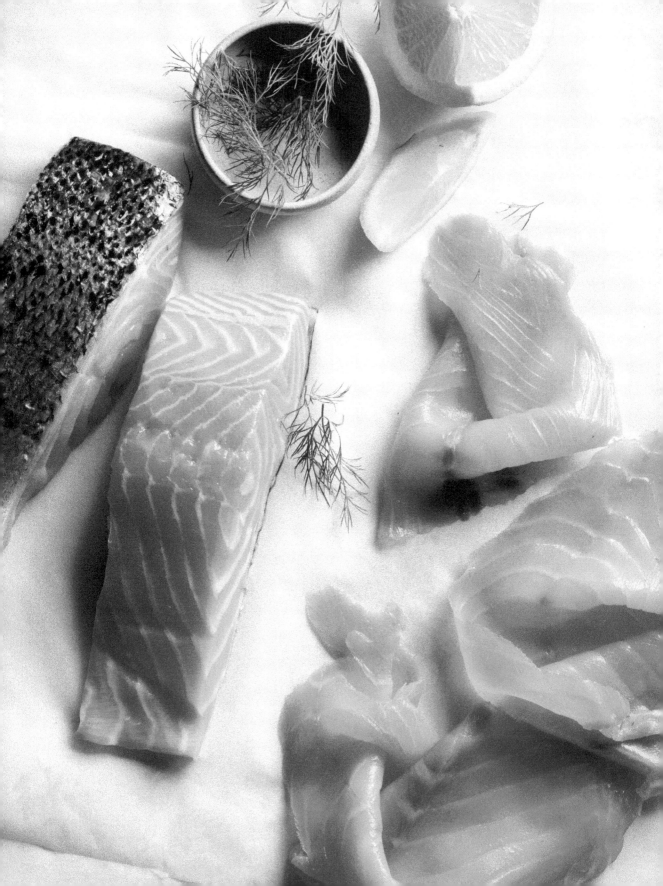

3

YOUR 28-DAY WEIGHT-LOSS PLAN

The meal plans that follow are specifically designed for those over 50 looking to lose weight following a low-carb, high–healthy fat ketogenic diet while using the tasty recipes in this book. Each day across the four weeks includes breakfast, lunch, a snack, and dinner as well as suggested daily exercise. The snacks are optional. You may find yourself feeling more satiated with the higher-fat meals, and as you come off carb and sugar cravings, you may not find yourself hungry between meals. If you are not in need of the snack, do not include it as learning to listen to your body's hunger cues is part of making this process a true lifestyle. Similarly, you may find that, over time, you are more comfortable with just two meals a day with or without a snack. If this is the case, breakfast is typically the smallest meal each day and an easy one to drop if you are ready to do so.

Each week has a full grocery list with all the ingredients you will need to make the recipes for that week. The weeks build upon each other and many of the upfront ingredients you will need, such as sugar-free sweetener (if using), almond flour, nuts, seeds, and spices, are used across the four weeks. However, I have included these ingredients in the shopping lists should you start with the weeks out of order. Each week also has a prep-ahead guide to help you make the most of your meal prep time at the start of the week. I also indicate where a recipe may be used as a leftover from the previous week.

Feeding More

Each of the four weekly plans is set up to feed just one person and minimize prep and cooking time each week. For this reason, the plans rely heavily on the use of make-ahead breakfasts and lunches, leftovers of main entrées, and repurposing ingredients. If you are feeding more than one or prefer less repetition in your meals, you may want to include additional main course recipes throughout each week. For those who love to cook and desire more variety when feeding just one, I encourage you to freeze half of each entrée to have for later weeks and incorporate more dinner recipes throughout the week, adjusting the shopping lists accordingly. I have made notes in each of the prep-ahead sections as to which recipes freeze nicely for this purpose.

Making Substitutions

Don't forget, flexibility and making this new lifestyle fit your preferences and schedule are important. Many recipes have substitution ideas in the tips section to offer ideas to change up flavors or ingredients to fit your dietary preferences. For example, if a recipe calls for pork and you don't consume pork products, substitute chicken or fish without compromising flavor or nutrition.

WEEK 1 MEAL PLAN

	BREAKFAST	LUNCH	SNACK	DINNER	EXERCISE
MONDAY	Broccoli and Cheddar Egg Casserole (page 54)	Curried Tuna Salad (page 94) with celery sticks	Chocolate-Almond Chia Pudding (page 128)	Ground Turkey Taco Soup (page 96) with Avocado Salad (page 133)	Cardio (see page 158), ideally in the morning
TUESDAY	*Leftover Broccoli and Cheddar Egg Casserole*	*Leftover Ground Turkey Taco Soup*	½ avocado with salt and pepper	*Leftover Curried Tuna Salad* with *Avocado Salad*	Strength (see page 160)
WEDNESDAY	*Leftover Broccoli and Cheddar Egg Casserole*	*Ground Turkey Taco Soup*	*Leftover Chocolate-Almond Chia Pudding*	Spinach and Goat Cheese–Stuffed Pork Tenderloin (page 110) with 2 cups mixed greens and 2 tablespoons Tangy Blue Cheese Dressing (page 153)	Rest day
THURSDAY	N'Oatmeal (page 57)	*Leftover Broccoli and Cheddar Egg Casserole* with 2 cups mixed greens and 2 tablespoons *Tangy Blue Cheese Dressing*	1 tablespoon unsweetened almond butter with celery sticks	*Leftover Taco Soup* with *Leftover Avocado Salad*	Cardio (see page 158), ideally in the morning
FRIDAY	Almond Joy Smoothie (page 52)	*Leftover Spinach and Goat Cheese–Stuffed Pork Tenderloin*	*Leftover Chocolate-Almond Chia Pudding*	Steak and Blue Cheese Salad (page 123)	Stretching (see page 162)
SATURDAY	*Leftover N'Oatmeal*	*Leftover Steak and Blue Cheese Salad*	10 kalamata olives	*Leftover Spinach and Goat Cheese–Stuffed Pork Tenderloin*	Cardio (see page 158)
SUNDAY	*Leftover Almond Joy Smoothie*	Double portion (4 halves) Guacamole Deviled Eggs (page 138)	*Leftover Chocolate-Almond Chia Pudding*	*Leftover Spinach and Goat Cheese–Stuffed Pork Tenderloin* with 2 cups mixed greens and 2 tablespoons *Tangy Blue Cheese Dressing*	Rest day

Week 1 Shopping List

PRODUCE

- ☐ Arugula, baby (4 cups)
- ☐ Avocados, medium, ripe (6)
- ☐ Broccoli, florets (2 cups)
- ☐ Celery (1 bunch)
- ☐ Cilantro (2 bunches)
- ☐ Lemon (1)
- ☐ Mixed greens (6 cups)

- ☐ Onions:
  - ☐ Red (2)
  - ☐ Yellow or white, medium (1)
- ☐ Peppers:
  - ☐ Bell, red (1)
  - ☐ Jalapeño (1; optional)

DAIRY AND EGGS

- ☐ Almond milk, unsweetened (½ gallon)
- ☐ Blue cheese, crumbled (4 ounces)
- ☐ Buttermilk (¼ cup)
- ☐ Cheddar cheese, shredded (½ cup)

- ☐ Cream, full-fat (1 [8-ounce] package)
- ☐ Eggs, hard-boiled (4)
- ☐ Eggs, large (6)
- ☐ Goat cheese (4 ounces)
- ☐ Sour cream, full-fat (¼ cup)

MEAT AND SEAFOOD

- ☐ Pork, tenderloin (1 to 1½ pounds)
- ☐ Steak, New York strip (6 ounces)

- ☐ Turkey, ground, not lean (1 pound)

FROZEN

- ☐ Spinach (1 [6- to 8-ounce] bag)

HERBS AND SPICES

- ☐ Black pepper, freshly ground
- ☐ Cinnamon, ground, or pumpkin pie spice
- ☐ Curry powder
- ☐ Extract, almond or vanilla
- ☐ Garlic powder
- ☐ Onion powder
- ☐ Salt
- ☐ Taco seasoning, reduced-sodium (1 [1-ounce] packet)

PANTRY

- ☐ Almond butter, unsweetened (9 tablespoons)
- ☐ Avocado oil
- ☐ Chia seeds (½ cup)
- ☐ Cocoa powder, unsweetened (3 tablespoons)
- ☐ Coconut milk, full-fat (2 [13.5-ounce] cans)
- ☐ Coconut, unsweetened flakes (¼ cup)
- ☐ Flaxseed, ground (2 tablespoons)
- ☐ Flour, almond
- ☐ Hemp hearts (¼ cup)
- ☐ Mayonnaise (6 tablespoons)
- ☐ Mustard, Dijon (1 tablespoon)
- ☐ Olive oil, extra-virgin (1½ cups)
- ☐ Olives, kalamata (18)
- ☐ Stevia, granulated
- ☐ Stevia, liquid
- ☐ Stock, chicken (16 ounces)
- ☐ Sugar-free sweetener (optional)
- ☐ Sun-dried tomatoes, olive oil–packed (4 ounces)
- ☐ Tomatoes, diced and green chilies (1 [10-ounce] can; preferably Ro-Tel brand)
- ☐ Tuna, olive oil–packed (2 [4-ounce] cans)

Prep Ahead

- Make the Broccoli and Cheddar Egg Casserole (page 54) to have for breakfast during the week.

- Make the Curried Tuna Salad (page 94).

- Make the Chocolate-Almond Chia Pudding (page 128) to have as a snack option. Leftover puddings will freeze if you do not need a snack.

- Make the Ground Turkey Taco Soup (page 96).

- Make the Tangy Blue Cheese Dressing (page 153) to have for the week.

- Make the filling for the Spinach and Goat Cheese–Stuffed Pork Tenderloin (page 110) and store, covered, in the refrigerator until ready to stuff and bake Wednesday night. Wrap 2 portions of the cooked pork tightly in aluminum foil and freeze for later (you will only use 4 of the 6 servings this week).

- The N'Oatmeal (page 57) can be made Wednesday night while the pork bakes to have ready for breakfast Thursday morning.

WEEK 2 MEAL PLAN

	BREAKFAST	LUNCH	SNACK	DINNER	EXERCISE
MONDAY	Carrot and Walnut Muffins (page 62)	Rotisserie Chicken Waldorf Salad (page 98) over 2 cups mixed greens	1 serving *Leftover Guacamole Deviled Eggs* (from Week 1)	Easiest Eggplant Parmesan (page 78)	Cardio (see page 158), ideally in the morning
TUESDAY	*Leftover Carrot and Walnut Muffins*	*Leftover Rotisserie Chicken Waldorf Salad*	1 serving *Leftover Guacamole Deviled Eggs*	*Leftover Easiest Eggplant Parmesan* with 2 cups mixed greens and 2 tablespoons Creamy Caesar Dressing (page 154)	Strength (see page 160)
WEDNESDAY	Cherries Jubilee Yogurt Parfait (page 59)	*Leftover Rotisserie Chicken Waldorf Salad* on Everything but the Carb Bread (page 150)	2 tablespoons nuts	Crispy Coconut Cod (page 93) with Italian Green Bean Salad (page 134)	Rest day
THURSDAY	*Leftover Carrot and Walnut Muffins*	*Leftover Easiest Eggplant Parmesan*	2 tablespoons nuts	*Leftover Rotisserie Chicken Waldorf Salad* on *Everything but the Carb Bread*	Cardio (see page 158), ideally in the morning
FRIDAY	*Leftover Carrot and Walnut Muffins*	*Leftover Easiest Eggplant Parmesan*	¼ cup full-fat plain Greek yogurt and 1 tablespoon unsweetened coconut flakes	*Leftover Crispy Coconut Cod* with *Leftover Italian Green Bean Salad*	Stretching (see page 162)
SATURDAY	*Leftover Cherries Jubilee Yogurt Parfait*	*Leftover Crispy Coconut Cod* with 2 cups mixed greens and 2 tablespoons *Creamy Caesar Dressing*	2 tablespoons nuts	Sausage Ball Soup (page 121)	Cardio (see page 158) followed by Strength (see page 160)
SUNDAY	Mediterranean Scramble (page 60)	*Leftover Sausage Ball Soup*	¼ cup full-fat plain Greek yogurt and 1 tablespoon unsweetened coconut flakes	*Leftover Crispy Coconut Cod* with *Leftover Italian Green Bean Salad*	Rest day

Week 2 Shopping List

PRODUCE

- [ ] Apple, Granny Smith, small (1)
- [ ] Basil (1 large bunch; optional)
- [ ] Carrot, shredded (1 cup)
- [ ] Celery (1 bunch)
- [ ] Eggplant, medium (1)
- [ ] Garlic (1 head)
- [ ] Green beans (1 pound)
- [ ] Kale, torn, or spinach (4 cups)
- [ ] Lemons (2)
- [ ] Mixed greens (6 cups)
- [ ] Onions:
  - [ ] Red (1)
  - [ ] Yellow or white, medium (1)
- [ ] Oranges (2)
- [ ] Spinach (1 cup, or ½ cup frozen)
- [ ] Tomatoes, cherry (6)

DAIRY AND EGGS

- [ ] Cheddar cheese, shredded (1 cup)
- [ ] Cream cheese, full-fat (1 [8-ounce] package)
- [ ] Cream, heavy whipping, or coconut milk, full-fat (2 tablespoons)
- [ ] Eggs, large (7)
- [ ] Feta, crumbled (2 ounces)
- [ ] Mozzarella, shredded (1 cup)
- [ ] Parmesan, shredded (1 cup)
- [ ] Yogurt, full-fat plain Greek (1¾ cups)

MEAT AND SEAFOOD

- [ ] Chicken, rotisserie (1)
- [ ] Cod, fillet (1 pound)
- [ ] Sausage, bulk Italian (1 pound)

FROZEN

- [ ] Cherries, dark (6)
- [ ] Spinach (1 [10- to 12-ounce] bag)

HERBS AND SPICES

- ☐ Black pepper, freshly ground
- ☐ Cinnamon, ground
- ☐ Everything bagel seasoning
- ☐ Garlic powder
- ☐ Ginger, ground
- ☐ Italian seasoning, or dried basil, oregano, or rosemary

- ☐ Onion powder
- ☐ Red pepper flakes
- ☐ Salt
- ☐ Tarragon, dried (optional)
- ☐ Vanilla extract

PANTRY

- ☐ Almonds, slivered (¼ cup)
- ☐ Anchovy paste (2 teaspoons; optional)
- ☐ Artichoke hearts, olive oil–packed (1 [4-ounce] jar)
- ☐ Baking powder
- ☐ Coconut, unsweetened flakes (½ cup plus 2 tablespoons)
- ☐ Coconut oil (½ cup)
- ☐ Cooking spray, nonstick
- ☐ Flaxseed, ground (¼ cup)
- ☐ Flour, almond (2¾ cups)
- ☐ Marinara sauce, no-sugar-added (1½ cups; preferably Rao's brand)

- ☐ Mayonnaise
- ☐ Mixed nuts (6 tablespoons)
- ☐ Mustard, Dijon (3 tablespoons)
- ☐ Olive oil, extra-virgin (¾ cup)
- ☐ Pecans, chopped (¼ cup)
- ☐ Stock, chicken (48 ounces)
- ☐ Sweetener, granulated sugar-free (10 tablespoons; Swerve or other brand)
- ☐ Vinegar, balsamic (2 tablespoons)
- ☐ Walnuts, chopped (1 cup)
- ☐ Worcestershire sauce

Prep Ahead

- Make the Carrot and Walnut Muffins (page 62). Cool completely and freeze all but 4 in a zip-top plastic bag for use another time.

- Make the Rotisserie Chicken Waldorf Salad (page 98).

- Make the Easiest Eggplant Parmesan (page 78) to reheat for dinner on Monday night.

- Make the Creamy Caesar Dressing (page 154) for using the next two weeks.

- Make the sausage balls for the Sausage Ball Soup (page 121) and freeze until ready to cook on Saturday night.

- Prep the vegetables for the Mediterranean Scramble (page 60) on Saturday night while the soup cooks to finish Sunday morning for breakfast.

WEEK 3 MEAL PLAN

	BREAKFAST	LUNCH	SNACK	DINNER	EXERCISE
MONDAY	*Leftover Mediterranean Scramble* (from Week 2)	*Leftover Sausage Ball Soup* (from Week 2)	Rosemary Nut and Olive Mix (page 130)	Salmon Alfredo with Zoodles (page 92)	Cardio (see page 158), ideally in the morning
TUESDAY	Breakfast Margherita Pizza (page 53)	*Leftover Salmon Alfredo with Zoodles*	*Leftover Rosemary Nut and Olive Mix*	*Leftover Sausage Ball Soup* (from week 2) with 2 cups mixed greens and 2 tablespoons *Creamy Caesar Dressing* (from Week 2)	Cardio (see page 158), ideally in the morning
WEDNESDAY	*Leftover Breakfast Margherita Pizza*	*Leftover Keto Chili* (page 124)	½ avocado with salt and pepper	*Leftover Salmon Alfredo with Zoodles*	Strength (see page 160)
THURSDAY	Cherries Jubilee Yogurt Parfait (page 59)	*Leftover Salmon Alfredo with Zoodles*	*Leftover Rosemary Nut and Olive Mix*	*Keto Chili* with 2 cups mixed greens and 2 tablespoons *Creamy Caesar Dressing* (from Week 2)	Cardio (see page 158), ideally in the morning
FRIDAY	*Leftover Breakfast Margherita Pizza*	*Leftover Keto Chili*	*Leftover Rosemary Nut and Olive Mix*	*Leftover Loaded Salad* (page 81) with 4 ounces pulled rotisserie chicken (optional)	Stretching (see page 162)
SATURDAY	*Leftover Breakfast Margherita Pizza*	*Leftover Loaded Salad* with 4 ounces pulled rotisserie chicken (optional)	½ avocado with salt and pepper	*Leftover Keto Chili*	Cardio (see page 158) followed by Strength (page 160)
SUNDAY	*Leftover Cherries Jubilee Yogurt Parfait*	Creamy Butternut Soup (page 82; will use leftovers in Week 4) with 2 ounces pulled rotisserie chicken (optional)	*Leftover Rosemary Nut and Olive Mix*	Korean-Style Barbecue Beef Lettuce Cups (page 118; will use leftovers in Week 4)	Rest day

Week 3 Shopping List

PRODUCE

- ☐ Arugula, baby, or spinach, baby (2 cups)
- ☐ Avocados, ripe (3)
- ☐ Butternut squash, cubed (2 cups, or 1 medium)
- ☐ Cilantro (1 bunch)
- ☐ Garlic (1 head)
- ☐ Ginger, paste (1 tube; or 2-inch piece fresh, or used ground)
- ☐ Lettuce, Bibb or romaine (1 or 2 heads)
- ☐ Lime (1)
- ☐ Mixed greens (8 cups)
- ☐ Onion, yellow or white medium (1)
- ☐ Oranges (2)
- ☐ Peppers, poblano, or green bell (2 medium)
- ☐ Rosemary (1 small bunch; or use dried)
- ☐ Sage (1 small bunch; or use dried)
- ☐ Spinach, baby (4 cups)
- ☐ Zucchini, spiralized zoodles (4 cups)

DAIRY AND EGGS

- ☐ Cream, heavy whipping (6 tablespoons)
- ☐ Eggs, hard-boiled (2)
- ☐ Eggs, large (4)
- ☐ Feta, crumbled (2 ounces)
- ☐ Mozzarella, fresh (4 ounces)
- ☐ Parmesan, shredded (¼ cup)
- ☐ Yogurt, full-fat plain Greek (1 cup)

MEAT AND SEAFOOD

- ☐ Ground beef (1 pound)
- ☐ Rotisserie chicken (1; optional)
- ☐ Salmon, fillet (1 pound; preferably wild-caught)
- ☐ Skirt steak (1 pound)

FROZEN

- [ ] Cherries, dark (6)

HERBS AND SPICES

- [ ] Black pepper, freshly ground
- [ ] Chili powder
- [ ] Cumin, ground
- [ ] Garlic powder
- [ ] Ginger, ground
- [ ] Oregano, dried
- [ ] Red pepper flakes
- [ ] Rosemary, dried
- [ ] Salt
- [ ] Vanilla extract

PANTRY

- [ ] Almonds, slivered (¼ cup)
- [ ] Beef stock (½ cup)
- [ ] Beef or chicken stock (32 ounces)
- [ ] Cashews (½ cup)
- [ ] Chilies, diced green (1 [4-ounce] can)
- [ ] Ketchup, sugar-free (½ cup)
- [ ] Marinara sauce, no-sugar-added (½ cup; preferably Rao's brand)
- [ ] Mixed nuts, unsalted (1 cup)
- [ ] Olive oil, extra-virgin (1¼ cups)
- [ ] Olives, kalamata (10)
- [ ] Pesto (½ cup)
- [ ] Roasted red bell peppers (1 [4-ounce] jar)
- [ ] Sesame oil (¼ cup)
- [ ] Soy sauce, low-sodium (¼ cup)
- [ ] Sriracha, or other hot sauce (optional)
- [ ] Sweetener, granulated sugar-free (such as Swerve; optional)
- [ ] Vegetable stock (16 ounces)
- [ ] Vinegar, balsamic (2 tablespoons)
- [ ] Water chestnuts (1 [8-ounce] can)

Prep Ahead

- Make the Rosemary Nut and Olive Mix (page 130).

- Make the Breakfast Margherita Pizza (page 53).

- The Keto Chili (page 124) can be made at the start of the week and frozen until ready to thaw for Wednesday's lunch.

- The Creamy Butternut Soup (page 82) can be made on Saturday to be reheated for Sunday lunch. It will be used in Week 3 as well.

WEEK 4 MEAL PLAN

	BREAKFAST	LUNCH	SNACK	DINNER	EXERCISE
MONDAY	*Leftover Carrot and Walnut Muffins* (from Week 2)	*Leftover Creamy Butternut Soup* (from Week 3)	Energy Balls (page 141)	*Leftover Korean-Style Barbecue Beef Lettuce Cups* (from Week 3)	Cardio (see page 158), ideally in the morning
TUESDAY	*Leftover Carrot and Walnut Muffins* (from Week 2)	*Leftover Korean-Style Barbecue Beef Lettuce Cups*	*Leftover Energy Balls*	*Leftover Creamy Butternut Soup* with *Curry Roasted Chicken Thighs* (page 105)	Cardio (see page 158), ideally in the morning
WEDNESDAY	Cherries Jubilee Yogurt Parfait (page 59)	*Leftover Korean-Style Barbecue Beef Lettuce Cups*	*Leftover Energy Balls*	*Leftover Creamy Butternut Soup* with *Dilled Cucumber Salad* (page 139)	Strength (see page 160) followed by Stretching (see page 162)
THURSDAY	*Leftover Carrot and Walnut Muffins* (from Week 2)	*Leftover Curry Roasted Chicken Thighs* with *Dilled Cucumber Salad*	*Leftover Energy Balls*	Mediterranean Snapper (page 90) with 2 cups mixed greens and 2 tablespoons *Creamy Caesar Dressing* (from Week 2)	Cardio (see page 158), ideally in the morning
FRIDAY	*Leftover Carrot and Walnut Muffins* (from Week 2)	*Leftover Curry Roasted Chicken Thighs* with *Dilled Cucumber Salad*	¼ cup full-fat plain Greek yogurt with 2 tablespoons slivered almonds	*Mediterranean Snapper* with 2 cups mixed greens and 2 tablespoons *Creamy Caesar Dressing* (from Week 2)	Stretching (see page 162)
SATURDAY	Southwest Scramble (page 58)	Cream of Broccoli Soup (page 143)	*Leftover Energy Balls*	*Curry Roasted Chicken Thighs* with *Dilled Cucumber Salad*	Cardio (see page 158) followed by Strength (see page 160)
SUNDAY	*Leftover Southwest Scramble*	*Leftover Cream of Broccoli Soup*	*Leftover Energy Balls*	*Leftover Mediterranean Snapper*	Stretching (see page 162)

Week 4 Shopping List

PRODUCE

- ☐ Avocado, medium (1)
- ☐ Broccoli florets (2 cups)
- ☐ Cucumber, English, large (1)
- ☐ Dill (1 bunch; or use dried)
- ☐ Garlic (1 head)
- ☐ Lemon (1)
- ☐ Mixed greens (4 cups)
- ☐ Onions, yellow or white, small (1), medium (1)
- ☐ Orange (1)
- ☐ Parsley, Italian (1 large bunch)
- ☐ Pepper, red bell, small (1)
- ☐ Tomatoes, cherry (16)

DAIRY AND EGGS

- ☐ Cheese, Cheddar, shredded (½ cup)
- ☐ Cream, heavy whipping (9 tablespoons)
- ☐ Eggs, large (3)
- ☐ Yogurt, full-fat plain Greek (¾ cup)

MEAT AND SEAFOOD

- ☐ Chicken, boneless, skinless thighs (1 pound)
- ☐ Red snapper fillet (1 pound)
- ☐ Sausage, bulk pork chorizo (4 ounces)

FROZEN

- ☐ Cherries, dark (3)

HERBS AND SPICES

- ☐ Black pepper, freshly ground
- ☐ Cinnamon, ground
- ☐ Curry powder
- ☐ Dill, dried
- ☐ Salt
- ☐ Thyme, dried
- ☐ Vanilla extract

PANTRY

- [ ] Almond butter, unsweetened (½ cup)
- [ ] Almonds, slivered (¼ cup)
- [ ] Balsamic vinegar (1 tablespoon)
- [ ] Chia seeds (1 tablespoon)
- [ ] Coconut, unsweetened flakes (2 tablespoons)
- [ ] Flour, almond (½ cup)

- [ ] Mayonnaise (¼ cup)
- [ ] Oil, olive, extra-virgin (1 cup)
- [ ] Olives, kalamata (30)
- [ ] Red wine vinegar (1 tablespoon)
- [ ] Stock, chicken or vegetable (32 ounces)
- [ ] Sweetener, sugar-free (optional)

Prep Ahead

- Pull out four Carrot and Walnut Muffins from the freezer (made Week 1) to have thawed for breakfasts this week.

- Make the Energy Balls (page 141).

- Make the Curry Roasted Chicken Thighs (page 105).

- Make the dressing for the Dilled Cucumber Salad (page 139) and wait to assemble the salad until Wednesday night.

- Make the Cream of Broccoli Soup (page 143) on Friday night or Saturday morning for lunch on Saturday and Sunday.

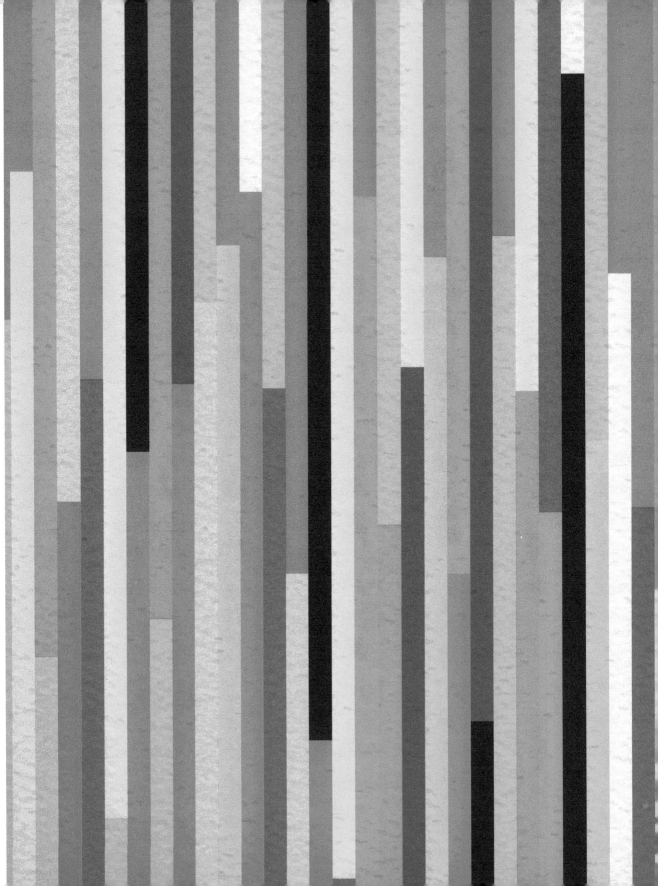

PART TWO

THE
RECIPES

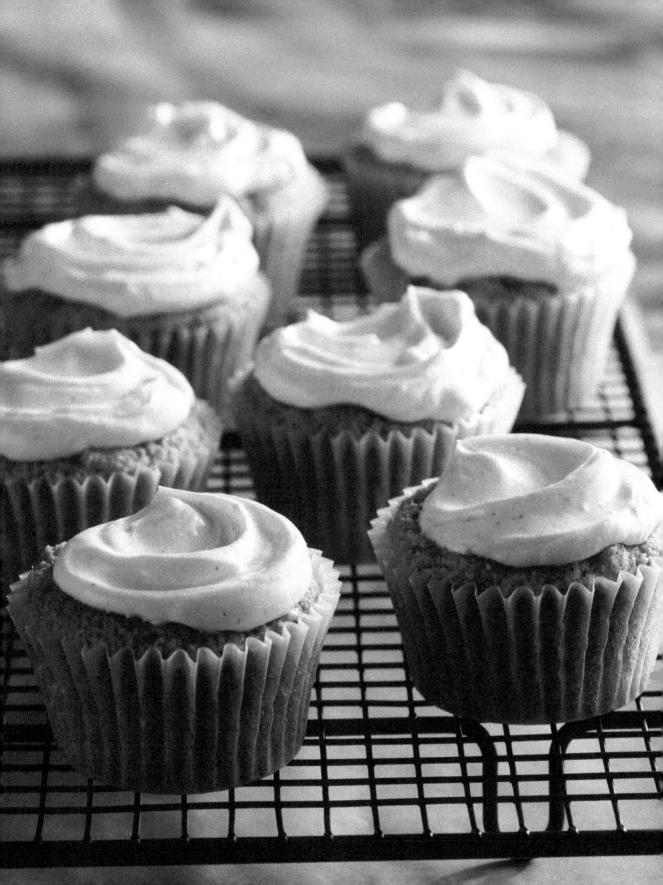

4

BREAKFASTS

Almond Joy Smoothie

Prep time: 5 minutes   **Serves 1**

With all the flavor of one of my all-time favorite candy bars, this nutritious and filling smoothie makes a great on-the-go breakfast for busy mornings. You can substitute any nut butter, such as cashew or peanut, for the almond butter, but be sure to look for versions with no added sugar.

1 cup canned full-fat coconut milk

½ cup unsweetened almond milk, plus more as needed

2 tablespoons unsweetened almond butter

1 tablespoon unsweetened cocoa powder

1 tablespoon unsweetened coconut flakes

1 to 2 teaspoons liquid stevia or other sugar-free sweetener (optional)

In a blender, combine the coconut milk, almond milk, almond butter, cocoa powder, coconut, and liquid stevia (if using) and blend until smooth and creamy, adding additional almond milk for a thinner consistency. Serve immediately.

Tip: For a slushier smoothie, add a handful of ice to the mixture before blending.

Per Serving: Calories: 662; Total fat: 64g; Protein: 12g; Total carbs: 23g; Fiber: 8g; Net carbs: 15g

Macros: Fat: 87%; Protein: 7%; Carbs: 6%

Breakfast Margherita Pizza

Prep time: 10 minutes / **Cook time:** 25 minutes   Serves 4

If you have trouble getting your veggies in the morning, this is the breakfast for you. This fun spin on eggs is loaded with micronutrients from the greens and quality protein and healthy fat from the eggs and olive oil. Add 4 ounces sliced pepperoni or cooked crumbled sausage for a heartier brunch meal.

¼ cup extra-virgin olive oil

4 large eggs

1 teaspoon salt

1 teaspoon dried oregano (optional)

1 teaspoon garlic powder

¼ teaspoon freshly ground black pepper

½ cup no-sugar-added marinara sauce (such as Rao's)

4 ounces fresh mozzarella cheese, cut into 8 thin slices, or 1 cup shredded mozzarella

2 cups arugula or chopped baby spinach

1. Preheat the oven to 375°F. Drizzle the oil into an 8- or 9-inch pie pan or glass baking dish and swirl to coat.

2. In a medium bowl, whisk the eggs, salt, oregano (if using), garlic powder, and pepper to blend. Transfer to the prepared pie pan.

3. Bake for 10 to 15 minutes, or until the eggs are just set. Remove from the oven, leaving the oven on.

4. Spread the marinara over the baked eggs and arrange the mozzarella slices on top. Top with the arugula, spreading it evenly. Return the pizza to the oven and bake for 6 to 8 minutes, or until the cheese melts and the greens wilt. Let rest for 5 minutes before slicing to serve.

5. Refrigerate the cooked pizza in an airtight container for up to 4 days.

Tip: Make a square pizza if you don't have a round dish by using an 8 × 8-inch square glass baking dish.

Per Serving: Calories: 306; Total fat: 28g; Protein: 11g; Total carbs: 3g; Fiber: <1g; Net carbs: 3g

Macros: Fat: 82%; Protein: 14%; Carbs: 4%

Broccoli and Cheddar Egg Casserole

Prep time: 10 minutes / **Cook time:** 35 minutes   Serves 4

I used to love making frittatas as the perfect egg-veg-cheese combo. As soon as I realized I could get all that flavor in an easier-to-prep and easier-to-reheat version, the casserole became my new go-to. Feel free to make this in a pie pan if you are a frittata die-hard traditionalist.

6 large eggs

1 teaspoon salt

1 teaspoon garlic powder

1 teaspoon onion powder

½ teaspoon freshly ground black pepper

½ cup shredded Cheddar cheese

4 tablespoons extra-virgin olive oil, divided

2 cups broccoli florets, large stems removed

2 tablespoons water

1. Preheat the oven to 375°F.

2. In a large bowl, whisk the eggs, salt, garlic powder, onion powder, and pepper to blend. Add the cheese and whisk until well combined. Set aside.

3. In a skillet over medium-high heat, heat 1 tablespoon of oil. Add the broccoli florets and sauté for 4 to 5 minutes until just browned. Pour in the water, cover the skillet, and remove it from the heat. Keep covered off the heat for 5 minutes, or until the broccoli is tender.

4. Coat the bottom and sides of an 8×8-inch glass baking dish with the remaining 3 tablespoons of oil.

5. Transfer the cooked broccoli to the egg and cheese mixture and whisk to combine. Pour the mixture into the prepared baking dish.

6. Bake for 20 to 25 minutes, or until the center is set completely. Serve warm.

7. Refrigerate leftover casserole in an airtight container for up to 4 days. Microwave to rewarm before serving.

> **Tip:** This is delicious with the addition of bacon or breakfast sausage. Simply cook 4 ounces of meat with the broccoli in step 3 and add it to the egg mixture in step 5.

Per Serving: Calories: 308; Total fat: 26g; Protein: 14g; Total carbs: 5g; Fiber: 2g; Net carbs: 3g

Macros: Fat: 76%; Protein: 18%; Carbs: 6%

Pumpkin-Pecan Muffins

Prep time: 10 minutes / **Cook time:** 20 minutes   **Makes 12 muffins**

Pumpkin, a starchy vegetable that is excluded on many ketogenic diets, is *loaded* with micronutrients including vitamins A and C, potassium, and fiber. Balancing the slightly higher carbs in this starchy veggie with healthy fats from the olive oil, almond flour, and pecans and extra protein from the eggs keeps them keto friendly.

4 large eggs

½ cup unsweetened pumpkin puree

⅓ cup granulated Swerve or other sugar-free sweetener

¼ cup extra-virgin olive oil or coconut oil, melted

1 teaspoon vanilla extract

1 teaspoon pumpkin pie spice

1¾ cups almond flour

¼ cup ground flaxseed

2 teaspoons baking powder

½ cup chopped pecans

1. Preheat the oven to 350°F. Line a 12-cup muffin tin with liners.

2. In a large bowl, whisk the eggs, pumpkin, sweetener, oil, vanilla, and pumpkin pie spice to blend.

3. Add the almond flour, flaxseed, and baking powder and mix until well incorporated. Stir in the pecans. Divide the batter evenly between the prepared muffin cups, filling each about three-quarters full.

4. Bake for 15 to 18 minutes, or until a tooth-pick inserted in the center of a muffin comes out clean.

5. Wrap leftover muffins individually in plastic wrap, then freeze in zip-top plastic bags for future use.

Tip: Vary the flavor by adding some orange zest and decreasing the sweetener to ¼ cup. Feel free to try other nuts, such as walnut or hazelnut, in place of the pecans.

Per Serving (1 muffin): Calories: 210; Total fat: 19g; Protein: 7g; Total carbs: 11g; Fiber: 3g; Net carbs: 3g

Macros: Fat: 81%; Protein: 13%; Carbs: 6%

N'Oatmeal

Prep time: 5 minutes / **Cook time:** 5 minutes **Serves 2**

Perfect on a cold morning, this hot porridge has all the comfort and flavor of classic oatmeal without all the carbs. The addition of quality protein and healthy fats makes this satiating dish a wonderful addition to a healthy ketogenic diet. If you've never had hemp hearts (hulled hemp seeds), you are not only in for a tasty treat, but also a nutrition boost: They are one of the only plant-based complete sources of protein, including all nine essential amino acids.

½ cup unsweetened almond milk or water

¼ cup hemp hearts

2 tablespoons almond flour

2 tablespoons unsweetened coconut flakes

2 tablespoons ground flaxseed

1 teaspoon ground cinnamon or pumpkin pie spice

1 to 2 teaspoons stevia or other sugar-free sweetener (optional)

1 teaspoon vanilla extract

1. In a small saucepan over high heat, whisk the almond milk, hemp hearts, almond flour, coconut flakes, flaxseed, cinnamon, stevia (if using), and vanilla to blend and bring to a boil. Reduce the heat to low and simmer for 3 to 4 minutes, whisking constantly, until thickened. Divide the N'oatmeal between 2 bowls and serve warm.

2. Refrigerate leftover N'oatmeal in an airtight container for up to 4 days. Stir in 1 to 2 tablespoons of almond milk or water before reheating in the microwave.

Tip: To prepare this in the microwave, combine all the ingredients in a microwave-safe bowl, stir well, and microwave on high power for 90 seconds. Remove, stir, and return to the microwave on high for 30 seconds. Serve warm.

Per Serving: Calories: 268; Total fat: 20g; Protein: 11g; Total carbs: 9g; Fiber: 6g; Net carbs: 3g

Macros: Fat: 67%; Protein: 16%; Carbs: 17%

Southwest Scramble

Prep time: 5 minutes / **Cook time:** 10 minutes   **Serves 2**

This simple scramble gets all its deep spicy flavor from chorizo, a pork sausage common in Latin American and Spanish cuisines, with just the right amount of heat. If you can't find chorizo, use hot Italian pork sausage.

3 large eggs

½ teaspoon salt

¼ teaspoon freshly ground black pepper

1 tablespoon extra-virgin olive oil

4 ounces raw pork chorizo sausage

6 cherry tomatoes, halved

1 medium avocado, peeled, pitted, and diced

1. In a medium bowl, whisk the eggs, salt, and pepper to blend.

2. In a medium skillet over medium heat, heat the oil. Add the chorizo and cook for 4 to 5 minutes, stirring frequently to break up any clumps, until browned and most of the fat has been rendered. Add the tomatoes and sauté for 1 minute.

3. Add the whisked eggs to the browned chorizo and scramble for 2 to 3 minutes, moving the eggs constantly in the skillet with a spatula to prevent sticking, until the eggs are cooked through. Remove from the heat and stir in the avocado. Divide the mixture between 2 plates and serve warm.

4. Refrigerate leftover scramble in an airtight container for up to 2 days. Reheat in the microwave, or return to a hot skillet to heat until warmed through.

Tip: If you want to make this ahead to reheat later, add the avocado after reheating the eggs and just before serving to prevent it from getting brown.

Per Serving: Calories: 467; Total fat: 40g; Protein: 19g; Total carbs: 11g; Fiber: 5g; Net carbs: 6g

Macros: Fat: 77%; Protein: 16%; Carbs: 7%

Cherries Jubilee Yogurt Parfait

Prep time: 5 minutes   **Serves 1**

Dark cherries are a wonderful superfood full of antioxidants that work to reduce inflammation and improve joint health. Here, a little goes a long way, and the cherries lend just enough sweetness, when combined with the orange zest and extract, that I find this parfait to be perfect without the addition of sugar-free sweetener. However, if you're slowly weaning yourself off super sweet foods, you may want to add 1 to 2 teaspoons of sweetener to the yogurt to taste.

½ cup full-fat plain Greek yogurt

3 frozen dark pitted cherries, thawed and chopped with their juices

1 tablespoon heavy (whipping) cream or full-fat coconut milk

2 teaspoons grated orange zest

½ teaspoon vanilla extract

2 tablespoons slivered almonds

In a small bowl, whisk the yogurt, cherries and their juices, heavy cream, orange zest, and vanilla to blend. Top with the almonds and serve immediately.

> **Tip:** To prep this in bulk for the week, double or quadruple the recipe. Leave the almonds off and refrigerate the yogurt in individual containers for up to 5 days, adding the almonds just before serving.

Per Serving: Calories: 254; Total fat: 17g; Protein: 14g; Total carbs: 11g; Fiber: 3g; Net carbs: 7g

Macros: Fat: 60%; Protein: 22%; Carbs: 18%

Mediterranean Scramble

Prep time: 5 minutes / **Cook time:** 10 minutes   **Serves 2**

This scramble makes a great weekend breakfast when you're not rushing out the door, or you can prep all the veggies ahead to scramble quickly with the eggs before heading out the door.

3 large eggs

1 teaspoon Italian seasoning (optional)

1 teaspoon garlic powder

½ teaspoon salt

¼ teaspoon freshly ground black pepper

3 tablespoons extra-virgin olive oil, divided

1 cup coarsely chopped fresh spinach, or ½ cup frozen spinach, thawed and drained

¼ cup chopped olive oil–packed artichoke hearts

6 cherry tomatoes, halved

2 ounces feta cheese, crumbled

1. In a medium bowl, whisk the eggs, Italian seasoning (if using), garlic powder, salt, and pepper to blend. Set aside.

2. In a medium skillet over medium heat, heat 1 tablespoon of oil. Add the spinach and sauté for 2 to 3 minutes until just wilted. Add the artichoke hearts and cherry tomatoes and sauté for 1 minute, or until the vegetables are just soft.

3. Add the whisked egg mixture to the vegetables and scramble for 2 to 3 minutes, moving the eggs constantly in the skillet with a spatula to prevent sticking, until the eggs are cooked through. Remove from the heat and stir in the feta. Divide the mixture between 2 plates and drizzle each with 1 tablespoon of the remaining oil. Serve warm.

4. Refrigerate leftover scramble in an airtight container for up to 2 days. Reheat in the microwave, or return to a hot skillet to heat until warmed through.

> **Tip:** This is fantastic with 2 ounces of chopped smoked salmon instead of the feta.

Per Serving: Calories: 404; Total fat: 36g; Protein: 15g; Total carbs: 7g; Fiber: 2g; Net carbs: 5g

Macros: Fat: 80%; Protein: 15%; Carbs: 5%

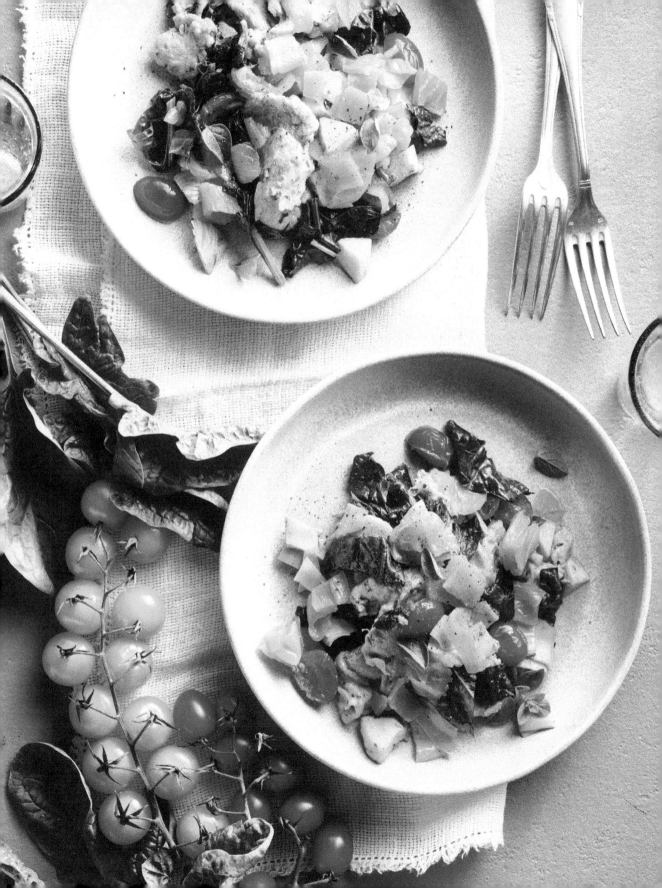

Carrot and Walnut Muffins

Prep time: 15 minutes / **Cook time:** 20 minutes **Makes 12 muffins**

These muffins are like having carrot cake for breakfast. This recipe makes a full dozen, and if you have trouble limiting yourself to just one as a serving, I suggest freezing what you don't plan to eat that week and pull out single servings as needed.

2 large eggs

½ cup, granulated sugar-free sweetener such as Swerve, plus 2 tablespoons

¼ cup coconut oil, melted

2 cups almond flour

2 teaspoons baking powder

½ teaspoon ground ginger

½ teaspoon ground cinnamon

1 cup shredded carrot

1 cup chopped walnuts

8 ounces full-fat cream cheese, at room temperature

1 tablespoon freshly squeezed lemon juice

1 teaspoon vanilla extract

1. Preheat the oven to 350°F. Line a 12-cup muffin tin with liners.

2. In a large bowl, whisk the eggs, ½ cup of sweetener, and coconut oil to blend. Add the almond flour, baking powder, ginger, and cinnamon and whisk until well incorporated. Stir in the carrot and walnuts. Divide the batter evenly between the prepared muffin cups, filling each about three-quarters full.

3. Bake for 18 to 20 minutes, or until a toothpick inserted in the center of a muffin comes out clean.

4. While the muffins bake, in a small bowl, whisk the cream cheese, remaining 2 tablespoons of sweetener, lemon juice, and vanilla until smooth.

5. When the muffins are done, let cool completely, then top each with 1 tablespoon of cream cheese frosting, spreading it evenly.

Tip: Freeze extra muffins in a zip-top plastic bag and individual (1-tablespoon) servings of the cream cheese topping in an ice cube tray or small plastic bags.

Per Serving (1 muffin): Calories: 296; Total fat: 28g; Protein: 8g; Total carbs: 18g; Fiber: 3g; Net carbs: 4g

Macros: Fat: 85%; Protein: 11%; Carbs: 4%

Green Eggs and Bacon

Prep time: 5 minutes / **Cook time:** 10 minutes ⬤ **Serves 2**

Dr. Seuss knew what he was talking about! These eggs get their green hue from pesto filled with heart-healthy olive oil and—what's better than ham?—crispy bacon. Add chopped fresh spinach or arugula for an extra green dose of micronutrients and fiber.

4 bacon slices

4 large eggs

**¼ cup jarred pesto
   or Versatile Pesto
   (page 149)**

**1 tablespoon
   extra-virgin olive oil**

1. Heat a medium nonstick skillet over medium-high heat. Cook the bacon for 6 to 8 minutes, turning as needed, until crispy.

2. While the bacon cooks, in a medium bowl, whisk the eggs and pesto to blend. Set aside.

3. Using tongs or a slotted spoon, remove the bacon from the pan, leaving the rendered fat. Add the oil to the rendered fat in the skillet.

4. Pour the egg mixture into the skillet, reduce the heat to medium-low, and scramble the eggs for 4 to 5 minutes, moving them constantly in the skillet with a spatula to prevent sticking, until cooked through. Serve the eggs warm with 2 bacon slices per portion on the side.

Tip: If using store-bought pesto, I prefer jarred pesto made with olive oil. If you can't find pesto, substitute 2 tablespoons olive oil, ¼ cup chopped fresh basil (or 1 tablespoon dried), and 1 tablespoon grated Parmesan, blended.

Per Serving: Calories: 521; Total fat: 47g; Protein: 21g; Total carbs: 6g; Fiber: 2g; Net carbs: 4g

Macros: Fat: 81%; Protein: 16%; Carbs: 3%

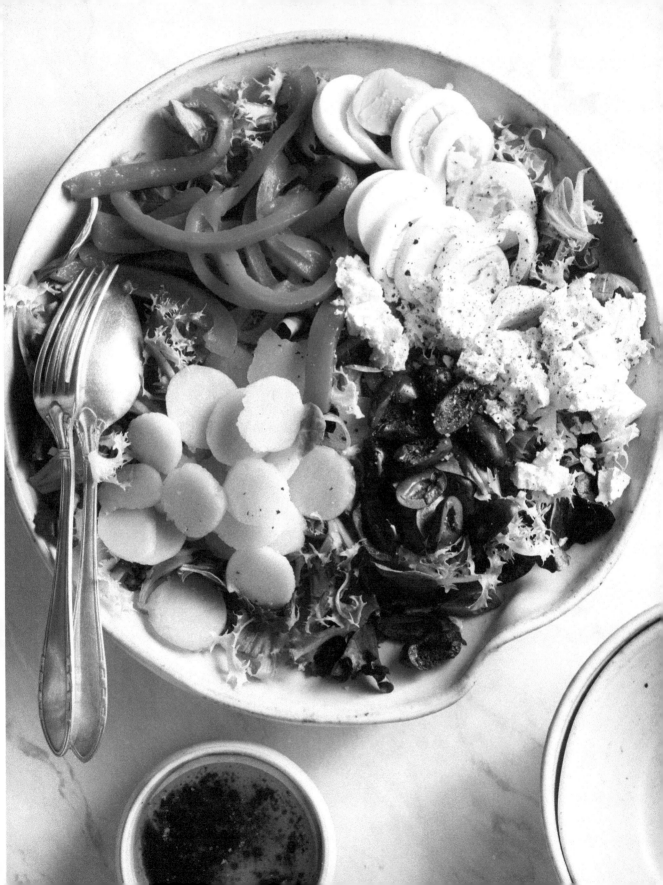

5

PLANT-BASED MAINS

Veggie-Loaded Cottage Pie

Prep time: 10 minutes / **Cook time:** 50 minutes   **Serves 4**

A traditional British and Scottish meal, cottage pie uses beef in the filling and is topped with a thick layer of carb-heavy mashed potatoes. This keto-friendly version doesn't skip on flavor or comfort and is full of micronutrient-dense veggies to keep it plant-based but uses mashed cauliflower to keep the carbs low. This serves four as a main or eight as a side to a simple grilled protein.

1½ cups cauliflower florets

½ cup shredded Parmesan cheese

2 tablespoons unsalted butter

1 teaspoon salt, divided

½ teaspoon freshly ground black pepper, divided

2 tablespoons extra-virgin olive oil

½ small yellow onion, diced

1 cup chopped red or green cabbage

1 carrot, peeled and diced

8 ounces mushrooms, diced

4 garlic cloves, minced, or 2 tablespoons jarred minced garlic

1 teaspoon dried thyme (optional)

4 cups chopped arugula or baby spinach

4 ounces full-fat cream cheese, at room temperature

1. Preheat the oven to 375°F.

2. Place the cauliflower in a steamer basket set over boiling water, cover the pot, and steam the cauliflower for 5 to 8 minutes, or until tender. Alternatively, place the cauliflower in a medium microwave-safe bowl, add 2 tablespoons water, cover with a paper towel, and microwave on high power for 2 minutes, or until tender. Drain the cauliflower and return it to the pot or bowl.

3. Add the Parmesan, butter, ½ teaspoon of salt, and ¼ teaspoon of pepper to the cauliflower and, using a handheld mixer or immersion blender, puree until very smooth, or mash with a potato masher or large fork until smooth.

4. In a medium saucepan or skillet over medium heat, heat the oil. Add the onion, cabbage, and carrot and sauté for 4 to 5 minutes, or until just tender. Add the mushrooms, garlic, and thyme (if using) and sauté for 2 to 3 minutes, or until the vegetables are very tender.

5. Add the arugula and sauté for 1 to 2 minutes until wilted. Stir in the cream cheese until melted and creamy. Transfer the vegetable mixture into an 8×8-inch glass baking dish or 9-inch pie pan. Spread the pureed cauliflower over the vegetables.

6. Bake for 20 to 25 minutes until golden.

7. Refrigerate leftovers in an airtight container for up to 4 days. To reheat, cover with aluminum foil and bake in a 375°F oven for 10 to 15 minutes, or until heated through.

Tip: To make this meal come together faster, substitute frozen mashed cauliflower for the florets, microwave, and stir in the cheese until thickened.

Per Serving: Calories: 299; Total fat: 25g; Protein: 9g; Total carbs: 11g; Fiber: 3g; Net carbs: 7g

Macros: Fat: 75%; Protein: 12%; Carbs: 13%

Peanut-Lime Zoodles with Tofu

Prep time: 10 minutes / **Cook time:** 10 minutes   Serves 4

This dish has all the flavor of your favorite takeout but with the nutrition and low-carb profile to make it work for your keto lifestyle. For a nonvegetarian meal, substitute shrimp, pork, or chicken for the tofu.

½ cup unsweetened peanut butter

¼ cup soy sauce

2 tablespoons toasted sesame oil

1 tablespoon ginger paste (optional)

Grated zest of 1 lime

Juice of 1 lime

1 teaspoon red pepper flakes (optional)

1 to 2 teaspoons granulated Swerve (optional)

2 tablespoons extra-virgin olive oil

1 red bell pepper, cored and thinly sliced

8 ounces mushrooms, sliced

8 ounces extra-firm tofu, drained and cut into ½-inch cubes

4 garlic cloves, minced,

4 cups spiralized zucchini noodles

1. In a small bowl, whisk the peanut butter, soy sauce, sesame oil, ginger paste (if using), lime zest, lime juice, red pepper flakes (if using), and sweetener (if using) to blend. Set aside.

2. In a large skillet over medium-high heat, heat the olive oil. Add the bell pepper and mushrooms and sauté for 4 to 5 minutes until just softened. Add the tofu and garlic and sauté for 2 to 3 minutes, or until tender. Remove from the heat and pour in the peanut butter sauce.

3. Add the spiralized zucchini and toss to coat. Serve warm.

4. Refrigerate leftovers in an airtight container for up to 4 days. Leftovers can be eaten cold or at room temperature, or reheat in the microwave on high power for 1 to 2 minutes, tossing halfway through the cooking time, being careful to not overcook the zoodles or they will become mushy.

Per Serving: Calories: 423; Total fat: 34g; Protein: 18g; Total carbs: 19g; Fiber: 5g; Net carbs: 14g

Macros: Fat: 72%; Protein: 17%; Carbs: 11%

Tofu and Veggie Scramble

Prep time: 10 minutes / **Cook time:** 15 minutes   **Serves 4**

This vegan version of scrambled eggs is so full of flavor, with just the right amount of spice. This dish may soon become your morning egg alternative. Don't skip draining the tofu for the best texture.

1 pound extra-firm tofu, drained

¼ cup extra-virgin olive oil

½ yellow onion, minced

1 red bell pepper, minced

4 ounces sliced mushrooms

2 garlic cloves, minced, or 1 tablespoon jarred minced garlic

2 tablespoons curry powder

2 cups baby spinach or arugula

1 ripe avocado, peeled, pitted, and chopped

1. Cut the tofu lengthwise into 4 pieces. Lay them flat on a stack of paper towels and let drain for 5 minutes, pressing down with additional dry paper towels to release excess water. Cut the drained tofu into chunks and place them in a large bowl. Using a fork, crumble the tofu into bite-size pieces.

2. In medium skillet over medium-high heat, heat the oil. Add the onion, bell pepper, and mushrooms and sauté for 3 to 4 minutes until the vegetables are tender. Add the garlic and sauté for 1 to 2 minutes until fragrant.

3. Add the crumbled tofu and curry powder to the skillet and sauté for 3 to 4 minutes until the tofu is browned and crispy and the vegetables are very tender. Remove from the heat, add the spinach, and toss to coat. Serve warm, garnished with the avocado.

4. Refrigerate leftover scramble in an airtight container for up to 4 days. Reheat in the microwave on high power for 1 to 2 minutes, or until heated through. If prepping ahead, add the avocado after reheating and just before serving.

Per Serving: Calories: 332; Total fat: 25g; Protein: 15g; Total carbs: 14g; Fiber: 7g; Net carbs: 7g

Macros: Fat: 68%; Protein: 18%; Carbs: 14%

Stuffed Portobellos

Prep time: 15 minutes / **Cook time:** 15 minutes — **Serves 4**

Goat cheese and sun-dried tomatoes add a whole new spin to this classic dish. I love these mushrooms as a plant-based main, or you can stuff the filling into smaller cremini mushrooms for an appetizer dish.

4 large portobello mushroom caps

3 tablespoons extra-virgin olive oil, divided

½ cup whole milk ricotta

4 ounces goat cheese, at room temperature

¼ cup chopped olive oil–packed sun-dried tomatoes, with their oil

¼ cup chopped fresh basil

½ teaspoon salt

¼ teaspoon freshly ground black pepper

1. Preheat the oven to 375°F.

2. Cut the stems off the portobellos and, using a spoon, scoop out the inner gills of each mushroom. Rub the inside and outside of each mushroom with 1½ teaspoons of oil (using 2 tablespoons total) and place them in an 8×8-inch or 9×13-inch glass baking dish, depending on the size of the mushrooms.

3. In a medium bowl, stir together the ricotta, goat cheese, sun-dried tomatoes and oil, basil, remaining 1 tablespoon of oil, salt, and pepper until smooth. Stuff one-quarter of the filling into each mushroom cap.

4. Bake for 10 to 15 minutes, or until the mushrooms are just tender but not mushy and the filling is heated throughout. Serve warm.

5. Tightly wrap leftover cooked mushrooms in aluminum foil and refrigerate for up to 4 days. Reheat, wrapped in the foil, in a 375°F oven for 4 to 5 minutes until warmed through, or without the foil in the microwave on high power for 1 to 2 minutes.

Per Serving: Calories: 276; Total fat: 23g; Protein: 11g; Total carbs: 8g; Fiber: 2g; Net carbs: 6g

Macros: Fat: 75%; Protein: 16%; Carbs: 9%

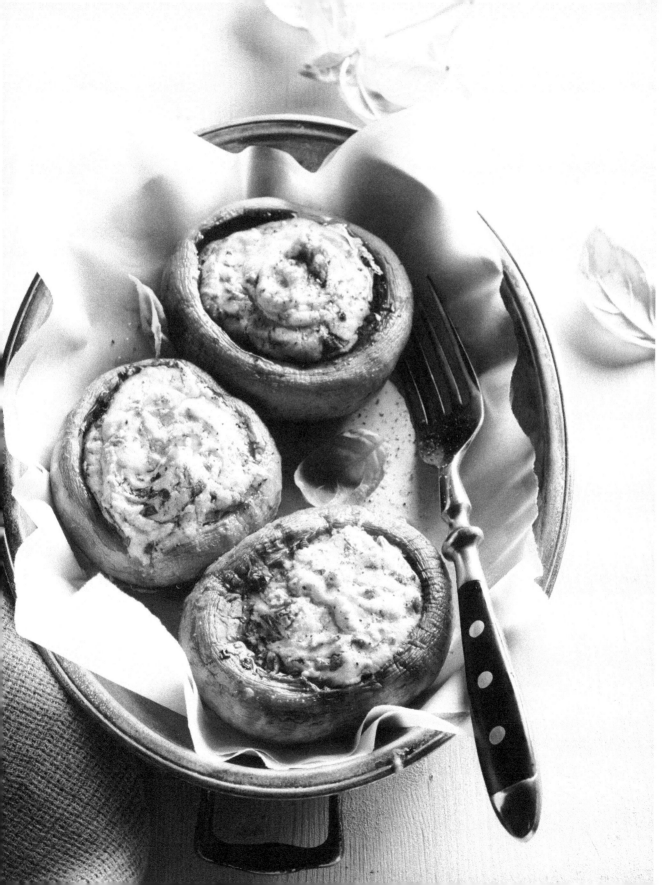

Walnut and Mushroom Burgers

Prep time: 10 minutes, plus 10 minutes to rest / **Cook time:** 15 minutes

Serves 4

These plant-based burgers get their wonderful savory flavor from the earthy flavors of sage, walnuts, and mushrooms. You can serve these burgers on their own with a simple side veggie or salad or wrapped in a lettuce leaf and topped with an avocado for an easy on-the-go meal. Using keto-friendly bread or a bun or the Everything but the Carb Bread (page 150) will increase calories significantly, so be careful if you are strictly adhering to your weight-loss goals.

½ small yellow onion, finely minced

8 ounces mushrooms, finely minced

1 cup finely minced walnuts

4 garlic cloves, minced

8 large fresh sage leaves, minced, or 2 tablespoons dried sage

1 large egg, beaten

2 tablespoons ground flaxseed

2 tablespoons almond flour, plus more as needed

1 teaspoon salt

½ teaspoon freshly ground black pepper

¼ cup extra-virgin olive oil

1. In a large bowl, combine the onion, mushrooms, walnuts, garlic, and sage. Add the egg, flaxseed, almond flour, salt, and pepper and mix until well blended. Let the mixture sit for 10 minutes to allow the vegetables and flour to absorb the egg and thicken.

2. Using your hands, form the walnut-mushroom mixture into 4 thick burgers, 3 to 4 inches in diameter. If you make the burgers too thin, they will fall apart.

3. In a large skillet over medium-high heat, heat the oil. Place the burgers in the hot oil. Cover the skillet and sear the burgers for 2 to 3 minutes per side, or until browned. Reduce the heat to medium and cook, covered, for 5 to 6 minutes, or until the burgers are cooked through. Serve warm.

4. Wrap leftover cooked burgers individually in aluminum foil and refrigerate for up to 4 days, or freeze for up to 3 months. Reheat in a skillet on the stovetop or microwave before serving.

> **Tip:** If you have a food processor, this recipe comes together in a breeze. Simply combine the onion, mushrooms, sage, garlic, and walnuts in the food processor and pulse until very finely minced. Let sit for 10 minutes, then transfer to a bowl and proceed with the recipe.

Per Serving: Calories: 332; Total fat: 31g; Protein: 9g; Total carbs: 9g; Fiber: 4g; Net carbs: 5g

Macros: Fat: 84%; Protein: 11%; Carbs: 5%

Tempeh and Veggie Curry

Prep time: 10 minutes / **Cook time:** 20 minutes   **Serves 4**

Tempeh is fermented soy protein full of nutty crunch and flavor. Not only is it high in protein for a complete plant-based meal, but the fermentation process also produces probiotics for a healthy gut and metabolic function. You'll find tempeh in most grocery stores next to the tofu in the refrigerated section, but feel free to substitute drained extra-firm tofu, if you prefer.

2 tablespoons coconut oil

1 small yellow onion, thinly sliced

1 red bell pepper, cut into ½-inch pieces

8 ounces mushrooms, sliced

2 tablespoons curry powder

4 garlic cloves, minced, or 2 tablespoons jarred minced garlic

½ teaspoon salt

1 (13.5-ounce) can full-fat coconut milk

4 cups baby spinach leaves, or 2 cups frozen spinach, thawed and drained

1 pound tempeh, cut into ½-inch-thick strips or crumbled

Cooked cauliflower rice, for serving (optional)

1. In a large stockpot over medium-high heat, melt the coconut oil. Add the onion, bell pepper, and mushrooms and sauté for 5 to 6 minutes, or until the vegetables are just tender.

2. Stir in the curry powder, garlic, and salt and sauté for 1 to 2 minutes until fragrant.

3. Pour in the coconut milk and bring to a simmer. Reduce the heat to low, add the spinach and tempeh, cover the pot, and cook for 5 minutes, or until the flavors are developed and the spinach is wilted. Serve warm on its own as a thick stew or over cauliflower rice (if using).

4. Refrigerate leftover curry in an airtight container for up to 4 days. Reheat in the microwave on high power for 1 to 2 minutes before serving.

Tip: If you're an eggplant fan, substitute 1 small eggplant, cut into ½-inch cubes, for the mushrooms for an equally low-carb and more traditional curry.

Per Serving: Calories: 489; Total fat: 37g; Protein: 28g; Total carbs: 22g; Fiber: 9g; Net carbs: 13g

Macros: Fat: 68%; Protein: 23%; Carbs: 9%

Shirataki Noodle Ramen Bowl

Prep time: 10 minutes / **Cook time:** 15 minutes   **Serves 4**

Made from the konjac plant, shirataki noodles have been eaten in Asia for more than 1,000 years. They are high in fiber and extremely low in carbohydrates, making them an optimal substitution for traditional pasta on a ketogenic diet.

4 cups vegetable stock

¼ cup toasted sesame oil

2 tablespoons miso paste or soy sauce

1 tablespoon ginger paste, or 1 teaspoon ground ginger

1 bunch baby bok choy, trimmed and thinly sliced

8 ounces mushrooms, sliced

2 garlic cloves, very thinly sliced

¼ to ½ teaspoon red pepper flakes (optional)

1 (7- to 8-ounce) package shirataki noodles (such as Miracle Noodle)

4 hard-boiled eggs, peeled and halved lengthwise

1. In a medium saucepan over high heat, whisk the stock, sesame oil, miso, and ginger paste to blend. Bring to a boil.

2. Add the bok choy, mushrooms, garlic, and red pepper flakes (if using). Reduce the heat to low, cover the pan, and simmer for 5 to 8 minutes until the vegetables are tender.

3. Add the shirataki noodles, re-cover the pan, and cook for 1 minute. Divide the soup evenly between 4 bowls. Add 2 hard-boiled egg halves to each bowl and serve warm.

4. To make ahead, keep the hard-boiled eggs separate from the cooked soup and add them just before serving. Refrigerate leftover soup in an airtight container for up to 4 days.

Tip: Baby bok choy can be found in the produce section of most grocery stores; substitute 2 cups thinly sliced cabbage if you can't find it.

Per Serving: Calories: 246; Total fat: 19g; Protein: 9g; Total carbs: 11g; Fiber: 3g; Net carbs: 7g

Macros: Fat: 70%; Protein: 15%; Carbs: 15%

Crispy Cauliflower with Coconut Cashew Cream

Just when you thought you were tired of this low-carb vegetable staple, this fun and flavorful way to dress up cauliflower will wow your taste buds. Roasting the cauliflower gives it a wonderfully crispy outside, and pairing it with the creamy sauce provides the best of both textures in one awesome dish.

2 cups cauliflower
  florets

2 tablespoons coconut
  oil, melted

1 tablespoon garam
  masala or Chinese
  five-spice powder

1 teaspoon salt,
  divided

½ cup canned full-fat
  coconut milk

¼ cup unsweetened
  cashew butter,
  almond butter, or
  peanut butter

2 tablespoons
  chopped cashews

1. Preheat the oven to 425°F. Line a rimmed sheet pan with aluminum foil.

2. Place the cauliflower florets on the prepared sheet pan. Drizzle with the coconut oil and sprinkle with the garam masala and ½ teaspoon of salt. Toss to coat, then spread the cauliflower into a single layer.

3. Roast for 20 to 25 minutes, depending on the size of the florets, until golden and crispy.

4. While the cauliflower roasts, prepare the cream sauce. In a small microwave-safe bowl, combine the coconut milk, cashew butter, and remaining ½ teaspoon of salt. Microwave on high power for 30 seconds. Remove from the microwave and whisk until smooth and creamy.

5. When the cauliflower is fully roasted, remove from the oven and drizzle with the coconut cream sauce, then toss to coat. Serve warm, garnished with the cashews.

6. If prepping this to eat later in the week, refrigerate the roasted cauliflower and cream sauce separately in airtight containers for up to 4 days. To reheat, roast the cauliflower in a 425°F oven until crispy and warmed through, and heat the sauce in the microwave on high power for 30 to 60 seconds until heated through. Toss to coat and serve warm.

Per Serving: Calories: 241; Total fat: 22g; Protein: 5g; Total carbs: 10g; Fiber: 2g; Net carbs: 8g

Macros: Fat: 82%; Protein: 8%; Carbs: 10%

Easiest Eggplant Parmesan

Prep time: 10 minutes / **Cook time:** 40 minutes   **Serves 4**

I love a good sheet pan meal for busy weeknight suppers. This simple keto-friendly version of an old favorite features hands-off cooking time and very little prep. You can double the ingredients to feed a crowd or have extras to freeze for another day.

2 tablespoons extra-virgin olive oil, divided

1 medium eggplant, cut into ½-inch-thick rounds

1 teaspoon salt

¼ teaspoon freshly ground black pepper

1 cup shredded Parmesan cheese, divided

1 cup frozen spinach, thawed and drained

1½ cups no-sugar-added marinara sauce (such as Rao's)

1 cup shredded mozzarella cheese

1. Preheat the oven to 400°F. Coat the bottom of a baking sheet or 9×13-inch glass baking dish with 1 tablespoon of oil.

2. Arrange the eggplant rounds in a single layer on the prepared baking sheet and drizzle with the remaining 1 tablespoon of oil, then season with salt and pepper.

3. Roast for 10 to 15 minutes until just tender.

4. Remove the eggplant from the oven and sprinkle with ½ cup of Parmesan. Return to the oven to roast for 5 to 10 minutes, or until the cheese is melted and golden.

5. Remove from the oven and top the eggplant with the spinach, marinara, and mozzarella, spreading the toppings evenly in layers. Sprinkle with the remaining ½ cup of Parmesan and return to the oven for 10 to 15 minutes, or until bubbly and the cheese is melted and golden brown. Serve warm.

6. Refrigerate leftover eggplant parmesan in an airtight container for up to 1 week, or freeze for up to 3 months. To reheat, thaw completely, cover with aluminum foil and heat in a 375°F oven for 10 to 15 minutes, or until heated through. Uncover and heat for 3 to 5 minutes more, or until the cheese is bubbly.

Tip: Let's face it: Not everyone loves eggplant as much as I do. Substitute zucchini rounds for the eggplant, if you prefer. You'll need about 2 large or 3 medium zucchini to cover the bottom of your pan.

Per Serving: Calories: 323; Total fat: 23g; Protein: 16g; Total carbs: 16g; Fiber: 6g; Net carbs: 10g

Macros: Fat: 64%; Protein: 20%; Carbs: 16%

Nutty Riced Cauliflower

Prep time: 15 minutes, plus 2 hours to chill (optional)

Cook time: 5 minutes   **Serves 4**

Cauliflower is a staple on a ketogenic diet as it makes a great substitute for many common carb-heavy sides, such as rice and potatoes. However, seasoned keto followers can get tired of the same old flavor profile, hence, this low-carb spin full of flavor and texture. I find that fresh riced cauliflower, made at home with a box grater or a food processor has superior texture. If you prefer to use a prepped version, seek out fresh rather than frozen prepared options.

2 tablespoons extra-virgin olive oil, divided

4 cups riced cauliflower (from about ½ medium head)

2 garlic cloves, minced, or 1 tablespoon jarred minced garlic

1 teaspoon salt

¼ teaspoon freshly ground black pepper

⅓ cup chopped fresh Italian parsley

¼ cup minced red onion

¼ cup chopped walnuts

¼ cup roasted pumpkin or sunflower seeds, hulled

Juice and grated zest of 1 lemon

1. In a large skillet over medium-high heat, heat 1 tablespoon of oil. Add the cauliflower, garlic, salt, and pepper and sauté for 3 to 4 minutes, or until tender but not mushy. Remove from the heat.

2. Stir in the parsley, red onion, walnuts, pumpkin seeds, the remaining 1 tablespoon of oil, the lemon juice and zest until well coated. Serve warm, or chill for 2 hours in the refrigerator, uncovered, to prevent the cauliflower from becoming mushy.

3. Refrigerate leftover salad in an airtight container for up to 3 days.

Tip: This salad is very versatile. Feel free to use another nut, such as almond or pecan, or change up the herb flavor using fresh mint, cilantro, or both.

Per Serving: Calories: 195; Total fat: 15g; Protein: 6g; Total carbs: 10g; Fiber: 4g; Net carbs: 6g

Macros: Fat: 69%; Protein: 12%; Carbs: 19%

Loaded Salad

Prep time: 15 minutes   **Serves 2**

This easy yet complete meal will kick up your salad making a notch. Water chestnuts are low in carbs and high in fiber, making them an ideal addition to any ketogenic diet for flavor and crunchy texture. The feta cheese is optional. If you want to omit it for a dairy-free version, increase the hard-boiled eggs to two per serving (four total) to meet adequate protein needs for a complete meal.

4 cups mixed greens

¼ cup thinly sliced jarred roasted red bell peppers

10 kalamata olives, pitted and halved

1 (8-ounce) can sliced water chestnuts, drained

2 ounces crumbled feta cheese (optional)

2 hard-boiled eggs, peeled and thinly sliced

¼ cup extra-virgin olive oil

2 tablespoons balsamic vinegar

½ teaspoon salt

¼ teaspoon freshly ground black pepper

1. In a large bowl, combine the mixed greens, roasted bell peppers, olives, water chestnuts, feta (if using), and eggs.

2. In a small bowl, whisk the oil, vinegar, salt, and pepper until blended. Drizzle the dressing over the salad and toss to coat. Divide the salad between 2 plates and serve immediately.

Tip: This salad can be prepped ahead in mason jars for quick lunches throughout the week. Make the dressing and add it to the jar first. Top with the salad ingredients, in layers, in this order: roasted bell pepper, olives, water chestnuts, feta (if using), greens, and eggs. Prepped salads will last in the refrigerator for up to 4 days.

Per Serving: Calories: 553; Total fat: 44g; Protein: 13g; Total carbs: 28g; Fiber: 6g; Net carbs: 22g

Macros: Fat: 72%; Protein: 9%; Carbs: 19%

Creamy Butternut Soup

Prep time: 15 minutes / **Cook time:** 35 minutes   Serves 4

This simple vegan soup is a favorite. The cashews provide a wonderful creamy texture without any dairy and are full of satiating healthy fats to make your body happy. Serve garnished with roasted pumpkin seeds or chopped avocado, if desired.

2 tablespoons extra-virgin olive oil

2 cups cubed peeled butternut squash

2 garlic cloves, minced, or 1 tablespoon jarred minced garlic

1 teaspoon salt, plus more as needed

¼ teaspoon freshly ground black pepper, plus more as needed

½ cup cashews

2 tablespoons chopped fresh sage, or 1 tablespoon dried

1 tablespoon ginger paste, or 1 teaspoon ground ginger

2 cups vegetable stock

1. In a medium saucepan over medium heat, heat the oil. Add the butternut squash, garlic, salt, and pepper and sauté for 5 minutes, or until the squash is just browned and fragrant.

2. Add the cashews, sage, and ginger paste and sauté for 2 minutes.

3. Pour in the stock, bring to a boil, reduce the heat to low, cover the pan, and simmer for 20 to 25 minutes, or until the squash and cashews are very soft. Remove from the heat.

4. Using an immersion blender, puree the soup until smooth and creamy. Alternatively, let the mixture cool slightly and transfer to a standard blender and blend until very smooth.

5. Serve the soup warm, seasoned to taste with more salt and pepper.

6. Refrigerate leftover soup in an airtight container for up to 4 days, or freeze for up to 3 months.

> **Tip:** You can find prepped cubed butternut squash in the fresh produce section of most grocery stores. Feel free to substitute frozen. If you prefer to use a whole squash, either peel and cube it or for more hands-off prep, halve the squash, remove the seeds, and roast it flesh-side down on an oiled baking sheet at 400°F for 20 to 25 minutes, or until softened. Simply scoop out 2 cups of cooked squash with a spoon and proceed from step 2.

Per Serving: Calories: 202; Total fat: 14g; Protein: 4g; Total carbs: 18g; Fiber: 4g; Net carbs: 14g

Macros: Fat: 62%; Protein: 8%; Carbs: 30%

Balsamic Baked Tofu

Prep time: 10 minutes / **Cook time:** 20 minutes, plus 24 hours to marinate (optional)   **Serves 4**

I like to keep this on hand to put atop a salad, toss into a refrigerator cleanout stir-fry, or even served on its own for a quick mid-afternoon snack. Many people are turned off by tofu, believing it to be bland and boring, but the flavors in this dish only get more intense as it marinates. I recommend letting it sit in the refrigerator for at least 24 hours before enjoying, although it can be eaten immediately after preparing.

2 teaspoons ground cumin

2 teaspoons smoked paprika

1 teaspoon garlic powder

1 (14-ounce) package extra-firm tofu, drained

⅓ cup extra-virgin olive oil

2 tablespoons soy sauce

2 tablespoons balsamic vinegar

1. Preheat the oven to 400°F. Line a baking sheet with parchment paper.

2. In a medium bowl, stir together the cumin, paprika, and garlic powder.

3. Cut the tofu into 4 large rectangles and place them on several layers of paper towels. Cover with additional dry paper towels and press down to release excess water. Cut the tofu rectangles into 1-inch cubes and transfer to the bowl with the spice mixture. Toss to coat well. Arrange the tofu cubes in a single layer, ½ inch apart, on the prepared baking sheet, reserving the bowl.

4. Bake the tofu for 15 to 20 minutes until crispy and golden.

5. While the tofu bakes, in the reserved bowl, whisk the oil, soy sauce, and vinegar until smooth.

6. Add the crispy tofu to the bowl with the dressing and toss to coat. Serve warm, or transfer to an airtight container and refrigerate for 24 hours.

> **Tip:** Change the flavor profile of this dish by altering the spices used. For a more Italian-inspired version, try dried rosemary and oregano in place of the cumin and paprika and replace the soy sauce with 1 teaspoon salt in the marinade.

Per Serving: Calories: 283; Total fat: 24g; Protein: 12g; Total carbs: 7g; Fiber: 2g; Net carbs: 5g

Macros: Fat: 76%; Protein: 17%; Carbs: 7%

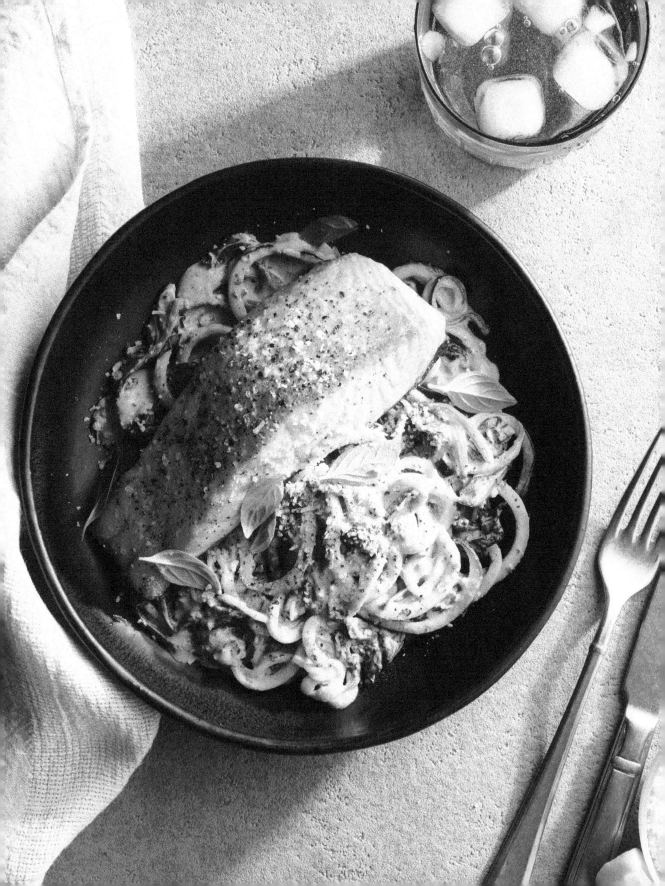

6

SEAFOOD AND POULTRY MAINS

Shrimp and Creamed Cauliflower

Prep time: 10 minutes / **Cook time:** 10 minutes — **Serves 4**

I'm from the South, and almost every Southern chef worth her weight in salt has a recipe for shrimp and grits. Decadent and full of simple flavor, this dish is a classic. Here, I've modified the grits base using low-carb creamed cauliflower but otherwise don't skimp on any of the flavor of the traditional favorite.

1 pound shrimp, peeled and deveined

1 tablespoon arrowroot (optional)

1½ teaspoons salt, divided

½ teaspoon freshly ground black pepper, divided

1 (8-ounce) package full-fat cream cheese

1 cup chicken stock, divided

2 cups fresh or frozen riced cauliflower, if frozen, thaw and drain off all moisture

½ cup shredded Cheddar cheese

2 tablespoons unsalted butter

½ small onion, minced

4 garlic cloves, minced, or 2 tablespoons jarred minced garlic

¼ cup chopped fresh Italian parsley (optional)

Hot sauce, for serving (optional)

1. In a large zip-top plastic bag, combine the shrimp, arrowroot (if using), 1 teaspoon of salt, and ¼ teaspoon of pepper. Seal the bag and shake to coat. Set aside.

2. In a medium saucepan, whisk the cream cheese, stock, remaining ½ teaspoon of salt, and remaining ¼ teaspoon of pepper to blend. Bring to a simmer over medium-high heat. Reduce the heat to low, add the cauliflower, and cook for 5 minutes, whisking occasionally, or until thickened. Remove from the heat and stir in the cheese.

3. While the cauliflower cooks, in a medium skillet over medium heat, melt the butter. Add the onion and sauté for 3 to 4 minutes, or until translucent. Add the coated shrimp and garlic and sauté for 3 to 4 minutes until the shrimp are pink and cooked through. Remove from the heat.

4. Divide the creamed cauliflower mixture evenly between 4 bowls. Top each with one-quarter of the shrimp mixture and garnish with the parsley (if using). Season to taste with hot sauce (if using) and serve warm.

5. Refrigerate leftover cauliflower and shrimp separately in airtight containers for up to 4 days.

> **Tip:** The arrowroot flour takes the place of cornstarch as a thickening agent to create a creamy thick gravy when the shrimp are cooked. If you don't have it, omit it in step 1 and just toss the shrimp with the salt and pepper.

Per Serving: Calories: 455; Total fat: 32g; Protein: 32g; Total carbs: 9g; Fiber: 2g; Net carbs: 7g

Macros: Fat: 63%; Protein: 28%; Carbs: 9%

Mediterranean Snapper

Prep time: 10 minutes / **Cook time:** 20 minutes   **Serves 4**

The vibrant, fresh flavor of the topping is what really shines in this dish. It works well with any flaky fish such as halibut, cod, or even salmon. Or, try it with a heartier steak-like fish such as swordfish or tuna. Simple but elegant, this dish will wow guests at a dinner party.

6 tablespoons extra-virgin olive oil, divided

1 pound red snapper fillet, cut into 4 (4-ounce) portions

1 teaspoon salt

½ teaspoon freshly ground black pepper

½ small yellow onion, minced

1 small red bell pepper, diced

8 garlic cloves, smashed

10 kalamata olives, pitted and halved

10 cherry tomatoes, halved

¼ cup chopped fresh Italian parsley

1 tablespoon balsamic vinegar

1. In a large skillet over high heat, heat 2 tablespoons of oil. Season the fish with the salt and pepper, place it in the skillet, skin-side up, and sear for 2 minutes. Flip the fish skin-side down and sear for 2 minutes. Remove from the skillet and keep warm.

2. Add the remaining 4 tablespoons of oil to the skillet, reduce the heat to medium, and add the onion and bell pepper. Sauté for 4 to 5 minutes, or until very tender. Add the garlic, olives, tomatoes, parsley, and vinegar and sauté for 3 to 4 minutes, or until all of the vegetables are very tender.

3. Return the fish to the skillet and spoon some of the vegetable mixture atop each fish portion. Reduce the heat to low, re-cover the skillet, and cook for 3 to 4 minutes, or until the fish is cooked through and flakes easily with a fork. Serve the fish warm with one-quarter of the vegetable-oil mixture spooned atop each fillet.

4. Refrigerate leftover fish in an airtight container for up to 3 days. Reheat in the microwave or serve cold atop a salad.

Per Serving: Calories: 346; Total fat: 25g; Protein: 23g; Total carbs: 8g; Fiber: 1g; Net carbs: 7g

Macros: Fat: 65%; Protein: 27%; Carbs: 8%

Creamy Dilled Salmon Salad

Prep time: 10 minutes, plus time to chill   **Serves 4**

So simple and refreshing, this salad makes a great lunch option or light dinner on a summer night. For a heartier meal, make an open-faced salmon melt using ½ Everything but the Carb Bread (page 150) and 1 slice Swiss or Cheddar cheese. Broil for 2 to 3 minutes to melt the cheese, and serve with a side salad.

¼ cup mayonnaise

Juice and grated zest of ½ lemon

2 tablespoons chopped capers (optional)

2 tablespoons minced red onion

1 tablespoon dried dill

½ teaspoon salt

¼ teaspoon freshly ground black pepper

1 (14-ounce) can salmon, bones and skin removed

1. In a medium bowl, whisk the mayonnaise, lemon juice and zest, capers (if using), red onion, dill, salt, and pepper to blend.

2. Add the salmon and combine well, breaking up any lumps with a fork. Serve chilled.

3. Store leftover salmon salad in an airtight container in the refrigerator for up to 4 days.

> **Tip:** You can used leftover cooked salmon in place of the canned, if you prefer. This salad is also delicious with canned tuna or chicken.

Per Serving: Calories: 224; Total fat: 15g; Protein: 22g; Total carbs: 1g; Fiber: <1g; Net carbs: 1g

Macros: Fat: 60%; Protein: 39%; Carbs: 1%

Salmon Alfredo with Zoodles

Prep time: 10 minutes / **Cook time:** 15 minutes   **Serves 4**

This dish may taste and look fancy, but it couldn't be easier with the help of jarred pesto and prepared zucchini noodles, found in the produce section of most grocery stores. I also love this made with shrimp or chicken in place of the salmon.

2 tablespoons extra-virgin olive oil

1 pound salmon fillet (preferably wild-caught), cut into 4 (4-ounce) portions

½ teaspoon salt

¼ teaspoon freshly ground black pepper

½ cup jarred pesto or Versatile Pesto (page 149)

¼ cup heavy (whipping) cream

4 cups baby spinach

4 cups spiralized zucchini noodles (zoodles)

¼ cup shredded Parmesan cheese

1. In a large skillet over medium-high heat, heat the oil. Season the salmon with the salt and pepper and add it to the skillet, skin-side up. Sear for 3 to 4 minutes, flip skin-side down, and sear for 4 to 5 minutes, or until cooked through and the fish flakes easily with a fork. Remove from the skillet and keep warm.

2. Add the pesto and heavy cream to the hot skillet and whisk until smooth. Reduce the heat to low and add the spinach. Cover the skillet and simmer for 3 to 4 minutes until the spinach wilts and the sauce is thick.

3. Place the zoodles in a large bowl and pour the hot sauce over the raw zoodles. Add the Parmesan and toss to coat. Divide the mixture evenly between 4 bowls and top each with a salmon fillet. Serve warm.

4. Refrigerate leftover salmon and zoodles in an airtight container for up to 4 days.

> **Tip:** For the best flavor and anti-inflammatory and heart-healthy omega-3 fats, look for pesto brands made with olive oil instead of canola oil.

Per Serving: Calories: 420; Total fat: 31g; Protein: 31g; Total carbs: 6g; Fiber: 2g; Net carbs: 4g

Macros: Fat: 66%; Protein: 30%; Carbs: 4%

Crispy Coconut Cod

Prep time: 15 minutes / **Cook time:** 20 minutes   **Serves 4**

Crispy and full of wonderful flavor, I love this dish served with a side of Cilantro Lime Crema (page 155) for dipping. The cod is also excellent atop a mixed greens salad tossed with Creamy Caesar Dressing (page 154).

4 tablespoons coconut oil, melted and divided

¼ cup almond flour

½ teaspoon salt

¼ teaspoon freshly ground black pepper

½ cup unsweetened coconut flakes

¼ cup ground flaxseed

1 large egg

1 pound cod fillet, skinned and cut into 4 equal pieces

1. Preheat the oven to 375°F. Line a baking sheet with aluminum foil and coat it with 2 tablespoons of coconut oil.

2. In a shallow bowl, stir together the almond flour, salt, and pepper. In a second shallow bowl, mix the coconut flakes and flaxseed. In a third shallow bowl, beat the egg.

3. One at a time, dredge each piece of cod in the almond flour, then the egg, and then the coconut-flaxseed mixture, to coat thoroughly. Place the coated fish on the prepared baking sheet. Drizzle with the remaining 2 tablespoons of coconut oil.

4. Bake for 15 to 18 minutes, or until the fish is golden and crispy. Serve the fish warm.

5. Refrigerate leftover cooked fish in an airtight container for up to 4 days, or freeze for up to 3 months. To retain the crispy texture, reheat in a 375°F oven for 4 to 5 minutes, or until heated through.

Per Serving: Calories: 374; Total fat: 29g; Protein: 26g; Total carbs: 6g; Fiber: 4g; Net carbs: 2g

Macros: Fat: 70%; Protein: 28%; Carbs: 2%

Curried Tuna Salad

Prep time: 5 minutes   **Serves 2**

The inclusion of curry powder in this simple recipe kicks the flavor up a notch from the average tuna salad and is soon to become a favorite easy weekend lunch option. If you're used to having tuna canned in water, you will be blown away by the rich flavor of the good stuff canned in olive oil. I prefer yellowfin tuna over albacore for both flavor and texture. Keeping leftover tuna salad on hand in the refrigerator makes a great afternoon snack if hunger strikes between meals. Serve cold on its own, atop a salad, or in a lettuce wrap.

2 tablespoons mayonnaise

2 tablespoons curry powder

1 tablespoon Dijon mustard

1 teaspoon garlic powder

1 teaspoon onion powder

2 (4-ounce) cans olive oil–packed tuna, undrained

2 tablespoons finely minced red onion (optional)

1. In a medium bowl, whisk the mayonnaise, curry powder, mustard, garlic powder, and onion powder until smooth and creamy.

2. Add the tuna and its juices and red onion (if using) to the mayonnaise mixture, using a fork to break up any lumps and combine evenly.

3. Refrigerate leftover tuna salad in an airtight container for up to 4 days.

Tip: I love using avocado oil mayo for both its flavor and heart-healthy anti-inflammatory fats. It can be pricey, so feel free to use any mayo you prefer.

Per Serving: Calories: 374; Total fat: 22g; Protein: 38g; Total carbs: 6g; Fiber: 4g; Net carbs: 2g

Macros: Fat: 53%; Protein: 41%; Carbs: 6%

Easy Chicken Vindaloo

Prep time: 10 minutes / **Cook time:** 25 minutes   **Serves 4**

A popular Indian-inspired curry dish, vindaloo traditionally requires slow cooking the meat in a thick cast-iron pot or tagine. Here, I cut the chicken into bite-size pieces to reduce cooking time and help this dish go from stovetop to the table in under 45 minutes.

¼ cup coconut oil

1 small onion, diced

1 pound boneless, skinless chicken thighs, cut into 1-inch pieces

4 garlic cloves, minced, or 2 tablespoons jarred minced garlic

1 tablespoon ground cumin

1 tablespoon paprika

1 tablespoon ground turmeric

1 tablespoon ground ginger

1 teaspoon ground cinnamon

1 teaspoon salt

½ teaspoon cayenne pepper or red pepper flakes (optional)

1 cup radishes, halved

1 cup canned full-fat coconut milk

½ cup no-sugar-added tomato sauce

Chopped fresh cilantro, for serving (optional)

1. In a large stockpot or saucepan over medium-high heat, melt the coconut oil. Add the onion and sauté for 4 to 5 minutes, or until tender.

2. Add the chicken and sauté for 4 to 5 minutes until browned on all sides. Add the garlic, cumin, paprika, turmeric, ginger, cinnamon, salt, and cayenne (if using) and sauté for 2 minutes.

3. Add the radishes, coconut milk, and tomato sauce and bring to a boil. Reduce the heat to low, cover the pot, and simmer for 10 to 15 minutes, or until the chicken is cooked through and the radishes are tender. Serve warm, garnished with cilantro (if using).

4. Refrigerate leftover chicken in an airtight container for up to 4 days, or freeze for up to 3 months.

Per Serving: Calories: 410; Total fat: 33g; Protein: 21g; Total carbs: 12g; Fiber: 3g; Net carbs: 9g

Macros: Fat: 72%; Protein: 20%; Carbs: 8%

Ground Turkey Taco Soup

Prep time: 10 minutes / **Cook time:** 25 minutes   Serves 4

Creamy and full of all your favorite taco flavors, this soup is perfect on a cold fall or winter day. I like this soup made with ground turkey, but you could use ground beef, chicken, or pork, if you prefer. Or, keep it vegetarian and add some spinach or mushrooms for extra bulk.

2 tablespoons extra-virgin olive oil

½ medium onion, diced

1 pound ground turkey (not lean)

1 (1-ounce) packet reduced-sodium taco seasoning

1 (10-ounce) can diced tomato and green chilies (preferably Ro-Tel brand), undrained

2 cups chicken stock

1 (8-ounce) package full-fat cream cheese

2 medium ripe avocados, peeled, pitted, and diced

½ cup chopped fresh cilantro (optional)

1. In a large saucepan or stockpot over medium-high heat, heat the oil. Add the onion and sauté for 3 to 4 minutes, or until softened.

2. Add the turkey and sauté for 4 to 5 minutes, or until beginning to brown.

3. Stir in the taco seasoning and tomatoes and green chilies with their juices and sauté for 4 to 5 minutes, or until the turkey is cooked through and fragrant.

4. Stir in the stock and cream cheese and bring the mixture to a boil. Reduce the heat to low, cover the pan, and simmer for 5 to 8 minutes, stirring occasionally, until the cheese is melted and smooth and the flavors have blended. Divide the mixture evenly into bowls and top each with one-quarter of the avocado and 2 tablespoons of cilantro (if using).

5. Refrigerate leftover soup in an airtight container for up to 4 days, or freeze for up to 3 months. Garnish with the avocado and cilantro after reheating and just before serving.

Tip: You can substitute plain diced tomatoes for the tomatoes and green chilies if you like a milder dish; use all green chiles for an even spicier version.

Per Serving: Calories: 717; Total fat: 57g; Protein: 36g; Total carbs: 18g; Fiber: 5g; Net carbs: 13g

Macros: Fat: 72%; Protein: 20%; Carbs: 8%

Rotisserie Chicken Waldorf Salad

Prep time: 10 minutes   **Serves 4**

This flavorful and crunchy chicken salad is a breeze to prepare. Apples are typically forbidden on a strict ketogenic diet due to their high sugar content. But here, a little apple goes a long way for crunch and flavor while keeping carbs low and ratios on point. You could substitute a firm pear for the apple, if you prefer, just keep the portion size to no more than ½ cup for the whole recipe. Serve the salad cold on its own, in Bibb lettuce leaves, or with Rosemary and Olive Oil Crackers (page 146).

¼ cup mayonnaise

¼ cup full-fat plain Greek yogurt

2 tablespoons Dijon mustard

1 teaspoon dried tarragon (optional)

1 teaspoon salt

¼ teaspoon freshly ground black pepper

2 cups chopped rotisserie chicken (about 1 pound)

½ cup diced celery

1 small Granny Smith apple, diced (about ½ cup)

¼ cup chopped pecans

1. In a medium bowl, whisk the mayonnaise, yogurt, mustard, tarragon (if using), salt, and pepper until smooth and creamy.

2. Add the chicken, celery, apple, and pecans and stir until well combined.

3. Refrigerate leftover salad in an airtight container for up to 4 days.

> **Tip:** Using rotisserie chicken makes this dish come together in a flash with minimal prep. If you prefer, use baked chicken thighs.

Per Serving: Calories: 380; Total fat: 26g; Protein: 34g; Total carbs: 5g; Fiber: 2g; Net carbs: 3g

Macros: Fat: 62%; Protein: 36%; Carbs: 2%

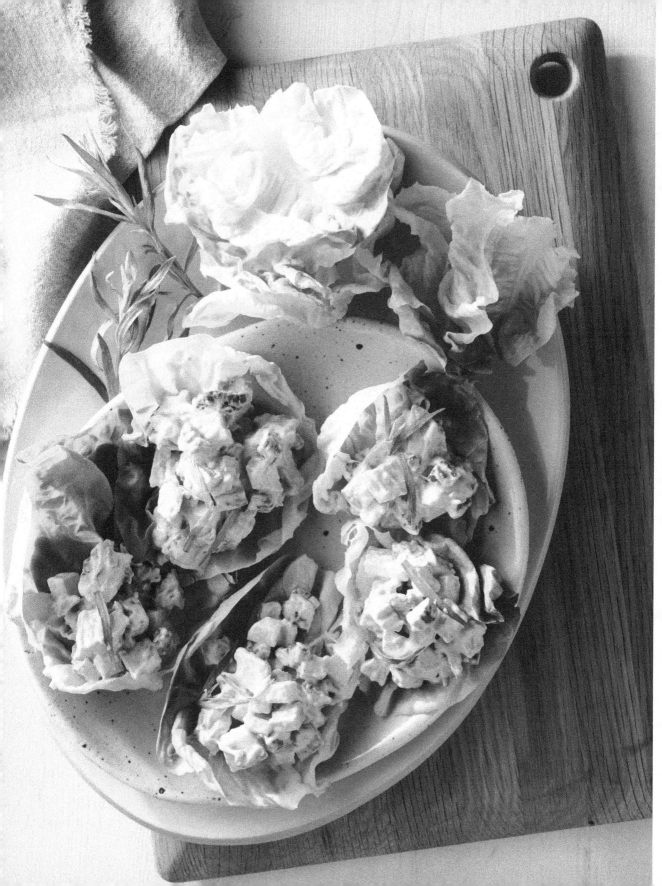

Chicken Lasagna Roll-Ups

Prep time: 10 minutes / **Cook time:** 40 minutes   Serves 4

My daughter came up with this recipe combining a few of her favorite dishes: lasagna, fettuccini Alfredo, and pesto chicken. What's not to love? This low-carb version uses zucchini slices in place of lasagna noodles to keep carbs low without sacrificing any of the other rich flavors and complexity of this creation.

Nonstick cooking spray or olive oil (optional)

2 medium zucchini, cut lengthwise into 8 (¼-inch-thick) slices

1 teaspoon salt, divided

1 cup shredded cooked chicken thighs (about 4 thighs)

½ cup jarred pesto or Versatile Pesto (page 149)

1 (15-ounce) jar no-sugar-added Alfredo sauce, divided, or Alfredo Sauce (page 156)

½ cup shredded mozzarella cheese, divided

1. Preheat the oven to 400°F. Line a baking sheet with parchment paper (if using aluminum foil, coat it with cooking spray or olive oil to prevent sticking).

2. Place the zucchini slices in a single layer on the prepared baking sheet. Sprinkle with ½ teaspoon of salt.

3. Roast the zucchini for 18 to 20 minutes until tender, but not crispy. Remove from the oven and let cool to the touch.

4. Reduce the oven temperature to 375°F.

5. While the zucchini roasts, in a medium bowl, combine the chicken, pesto, remaining ½ teaspoon of salt, ¼ cup of Alfredo sauce, and ¼ cup of mozzarella. Mix with a fork until the ingredients are well incorporated.

6. Pour half of the remaining Alfredo sauce (about ¾ cup) in the bottom of an 8×8-inch square glass baking dish.

7. To make the roll-ups, spread about 2 tablespoons of the chicken mixture halfway up each of the zucchini slices and roll up the slices starting from the chicken side. Place each roll-up in the prepared baking dish, seam-side down. Cover with the remaining Alfredo sauce and sprinkle with the remaining ¼ cup of cheese. Cover the dish with foil.

8. Bake for 15 to 18 minutes, or until the sauce is bubbly and the cheese is melted. Remove the foil and bake for 5 minutes, or until the cheese is browned. Serve warm.

9. Refrigerate leftover cooked rollups in an airtight container for up to 4 days. Reheat in a 375°F oven, covered in foil, for 8 to 10 minutes until warmed through and bubbly.

Tip: For easy shredded chicken, cook the thighs in boiling water or an Instant Pot or other electric pressure cooker until cooked through. Drain. Using a handheld mixer on high speed, shred the chicken.

Per Serving (2 roll-ups): Calories: 656; Total fat: 50g; Protein: 42g; Total carbs: 9g; Fiber: 1g; Net carbs: 8g

Macros: Fat: 69%; Protein: 26%; Carbs: 5%

Saucy Chicken and Mushroom Meatballs

Prep time: 15 minutes / **Cook time:** 30 minutes   **Serves 4**

These meatballs, in a thick, creamy, luscious mushroom sauce, are fantastic served over zucchini noodles, riced cauliflower, or a simple bed of sautéed spinach. I also love them served on their own with toothpicks as an appetizer or great party food.

2 tablespoons
extra-virgin olive oil

8 ounces sliced
mushrooms

1 pound ground
chicken (not lean)

½ cup grated
Parmesan cheese

1 large egg, beaten

4 garlic cloves, minced,
or 2 tablespoons
jarred minced garlic,
divided

2 tablespoons
chopped fresh Italian
parsley

1 teaspoon salt

¼ teaspoon freshly
ground black pepper

¾ cup chicken stock

¼ cup heavy
(whipping) cream

1 tablespoon
arrowroot

4 tablespoons (½ stick)
unsalted butter

½ small onion, thinly
sliced

1. Preheat the oven to 400°F. Line a baking sheet with aluminum foil and coat it with the olive oil.

2. Finely mince half of the mushrooms and place them in a large bowl. Add the chicken, Parmesan, egg, half of the garlic, the parsley, the salt, and the pepper and combine well. Using your hands, shape the mixture into 16 meatballs, about 1 inch in diameter, and place them on the prepared baking sheet.

3. Bake for 18 to 20 minutes, or until golden, cooked through, and no longer pink.

4. While the meatballs bake, in a small bowl, whisk the stock, cream, and arrowroot to combine. Set aside.

5. In a large skillet or saucepan over medium-low heat, melt the butter. Add the onion and remaining sliced mushrooms and sauté for 8 to 10 minutes, or until golden and translucent. Add the remaining garlic and sauté for 2 minutes until fragrant.

6. Whisk in the cream and stock mixture, bring to a boil, reduce the heat to low, cover the skillet, and keep warm until the meatballs are done.

7. Add the baked meatballs to the sauce. Re-cover the skillet and simmer for 3 to 4 minutes until the sauce is thickened. Serve the meatballs and sauce warm.

8. Refrigerate leftover meatballs and sauce in an airtight container for up to 4 days. Freeze baked meatballs (without the sauce) in a zip-top plastic bag for up to 3 months. Thaw, prepare the sauce, and add the thawed meatballs just before serving.

Per Serving: Calories: 529; Total fat: 41g; Protein: 35g; Total carbs: 8g; Fiber: 1g; Net carbs: 7g

Macros: Fat: 70%; Protein: 26%; Carbs: 4%

Chicken Margherita

Prep time: 10 minutes / **Cook time:** 25 minutes   Serves 4

All the classic flavors and gooey texture of your favorite fresh pizza without all the carbs. For an awesome pan pizza presentation, make this in a cast-iron skillet, finish under the broiler, and serve tableside right out of the skillet.

4 (4-ounce) boneless, skinless chicken thighs
½ teaspoon salt
¼ teaspoon freshly ground black pepper
2 tablespoons extra-virgin olive oil, divided
½ cup no-sugar-added marinara sauce (such as Rao's)
½ cup frozen spinach, thawed and drained
2 ounces fresh mozzarella cheese, cut into 4 (½-inch-thick) slices
4 to 8 large fresh basil leaves, thinly sliced

1. Season the chicken with the salt and pepper.

2. In a large skillet with a lid over medium-high heat, heat 1 tablespoon of oil. Add the chicken and brown for 3 to 4 minutes per side.

3. In a small bowl, stir together the marinara, remaining 1 tablespoon of oil, and spinach until smooth. Place ¼ cup of sauce atop each thigh and top each with 1 mozzarella slice. Cover the skillet, reduce the heat to low, and simmer for 8 to 10 minutes until the chicken is cooked through and the cheese melts.

4. Top with the basil leaves and serve warm.

5. Refrigerate leftover chicken in an airtight container for up to 4 days.

Tip: Nothing beats the intense flavor of fresh basil, but you can substitute 1 tablespoon Italian seasoning or dried basil.

Per Serving: Calories: 255; Total fat: 19g; Protein: 22g; Total carbs: 2g; Fiber: 1g; Net carbs: 1g

Macros: Fat: 67%; Protein: 33%; Carbs: <1%

Curry Roasted Chicken Thighs

Prep time: 5 minutes / **Cook time:** 35 minutes   Serves 4

This flavor-rich easy protein-filled dish is about as hands-off as home cooking gets. If you don't love curry, use any other favorite spice blend, such as Chinese five-spice powder, Italian seasoning, garam masala, za'atar, or Greek seasoning. You can roast asparagus, broccoli, or Brussels sprouts alongside the chicken as it bakes. Serve with the Cilantro Lime Crema (page 155) or Tzatziki (page 157) for a special treat.

1 pound boneless, skinless chicken thighs
¼ cup extra-virgin olive oil
2 tablespoons curry powder
1 teaspoon salt
1 lemon, cut into thin slices

1. Preheat the oven to 400°F.

2. In a large bowl, toss together the chicken, oil, curry powder, and salt. Transfer to a glass baking dish and top with the lemon slices. Cover the dish with aluminum foil.

3. Bake for 20 to 25 minutes, covered, or until the chicken is almost cooked throughout. Uncover and bake for 5 to 10 minutes, or until chicken is golden and cooked through and no longer pink.

4. Refrigerate leftover cooked chicken in an airtight container for up to 4 days.

Tip: You can double or triple this recipe to have extra on hand throughout the week. Chop and blend with mayonnaise and diced celery for an easy chicken salad or serve atop a mixed greens salad with avocado and roasted pumpkin seeds.

Per Serving: Calories: 264; Total fat: 21g; Protein: 19g; Total carbs: 3g; Fiber: 2g; Net carbs: 1g

Macros: Fat: 72%; Protein: 28%; Carbs: <1%

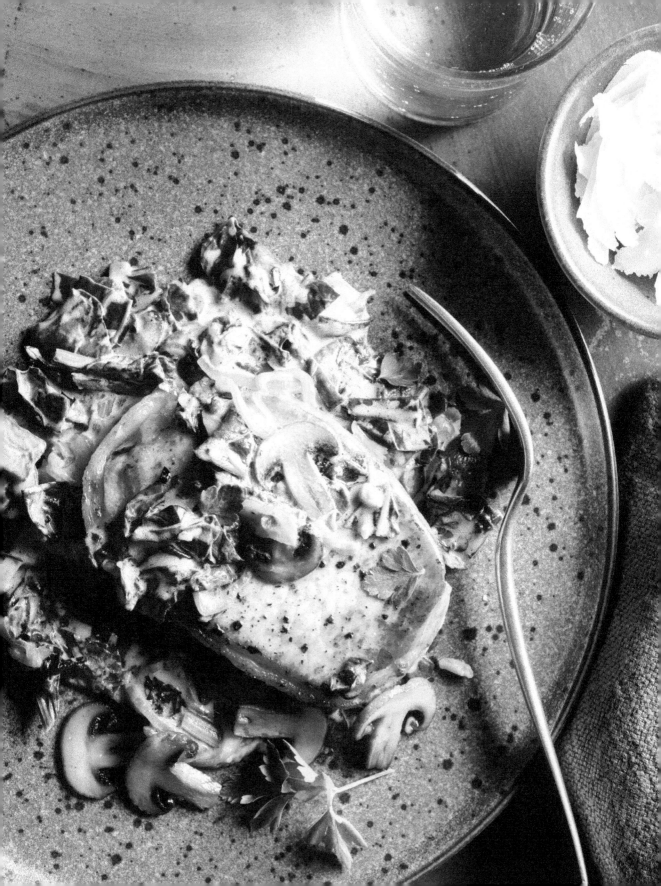

7

MEAT MAINS

Greek Meatballs

Prep time: 10 minutes / **Cook time:** 25 minutes   **Serves 4**

I adore the earthy flavor of lamb mixed with sweet and refreshing mint, but feel free to use ground beef, if you prefer. Serve these meatballs with a side of Tzatziki (page 157) and Dilled Cucumber Salad (page 139). Leftover meatballs can be served cold atop a Loaded Salad (page 81) for a satisfying lunch.

2 tablespoons extra-virgin olive oil

1 pound ground lamb

2 ounces crumbled feta cheese

½ cup packed coarsely chopped fresh mint leaves

¼ cup minced red onion

1 garlic clove, minced

1 teaspoon salt

¼ teaspoon freshly ground black pepper

1. Preheat the oven to 375°F. Line a baking sheet with aluminum foil and coat it with the oil.

2. In a large bowl, combine the lamb, feta, mint, red onion, garlic, salt, and pepper and mix to incorporate all ingredients. Using your hands, form the mixture into 16 meatballs, about 1 inch in diameter, and place them on the prepared baking sheet.

3. Bake for 20 to 25 minutes, or until browned. Serve warm.

4. Refrigerate leftover meatballs in an airtight container for up to 4 days, or freeze in a zip-top plastic bag for up to 3 months.

Tip: You can change up the flavor here but retain all the cheesy goodness by using Italian seasoning and chopped parsley in place of the mint and red onion.

Per Serving: Calories: 427; Total fat: 36g; Protein: 21g; Total carbs: 3g; Fiber: 1g; Net carbs: 2g

Macros: Fat: 76%; Protein: 20%; Carbs: 4%

Flank Steak with Mint Chimichurri

Prep time: 10 minutes / **Cook time:** 20 minutes  **Serves 4**

Full of herb and garlic flavor, chimichurri is served with just about any grilled protein, but mostly beef. Leftover chimichurri is also fantastic mixed with scrambled eggs or stirred into canned tuna for a quick lunch salad.

1 pound flank steak

2 tablespoons extra-virgin olive oil, plus ¼ cup

1½ teaspoons salt, divided

½ teaspoon freshly ground black pepper, divided

1 cup packed finely minced fresh mint leaves

4 garlic cloves, minced, or 2 tablespoons jarred minced garlic

Juice and grated zest of ½ orange

1. Preheat a grill to medium-high heat, or preheat the oven to 450°F.

2. Rub the steak with 2 tablespoons of oil and season with 1 teaspoon of salt and ¼ teaspoon of pepper. Let sit at room temperature while you make the sauce.

3. In a small bowl, whisk the remaining ¼ cup of oil, mint, garlic, orange juice and zest, remaining ½ teaspoon of salt, and remaining ¼ teaspoon of pepper to blend. Set aside.

4. Put the steak on the grill and cook for 6 to 8 minutes per side, or to your desired doneness. If using an oven, heat an oven-safe skillet (preferably cast iron) over high heat. Add the steak and sear for 1 to 2 minutes per side. Transfer the skillet to the oven and roast the steak for 8 to 10 minutes. Let rest for 5 minutes before slicing. Serve the steak warm, with each portion drizzled with 2 tablespoons of chimichurri.

5. Refrigerate leftover chimichurri in an airtight container for up to 2 weeks.

Per Serving: Calories: 398; Total fat: 31g; Protein: 25g; Total carbs: 4g; Fiber: 2g; Net carbs: 2g

Macros: Fat: 70%; Protein: 25%; Carbs: 5%

Spinach and Goat Cheese— Stuffed Pork Tenderloin

Prep time: 15 minutes / **Cook time:** 30 minutes   **Serves 6**

Anything made with creamy goat cheese is a win in my book. This simple yet decadent filling transforms a plain pork dish into a fancy dinner meal. Use the same technique to stuff pork chops or chicken breasts in place of the full tenderloin.

1 (1- to 1½-pound) pork tenderloin

6 tablespoons extra-virgin olive oil, divided

4 ounces goat cheese

⅔ cup frozen spinach, thawed and drained

¼ cup chopped olive oil–packed sun-dried tomatoes, with their oil

1 teaspoon salt

1 teaspoon garlic powder

¼ teaspoon freshly ground black pepper

1. Preheat the oven to 375°F.

2. Without cutting through to the other side, made a deep slit lengthwise along the tenderloin, leaving about 2 inches on each end to create a pocket. Using your fingers, carefully increase the size of the pocket.

3. Spread 2 tablespoons of olive oil over the outside of the tenderloin and inside the pocket. Place the tenderloin into a 9×13-inch glass baking dish.

4. In a medium bowl, stir together the goat cheese, spinach, sun-dried tomatoes and oil, remaining 4 tablespoons of olive oil, the salt, the garlic powder, and the pepper until well combined. Stuff the mixture into the tenderloin pocket and use your hands to press the opening together to seal it. Cover the dish with aluminum foil.

5. Bake for 20 to 25 minutes, depending on the size of the tenderloin, or until a meat thermometer inserted into the pork (not the filling) reads 155°F. Remove the foil and bake for 5 minutes to brown the outside. Remove from the

oven and let sit for 10 minutes before slicing. Serve warm.

6. Refrigerate leftover cooked pork in an airtight container for up to 4 days. Reheat in the micro-wave, or covered in foil in a 375°F oven for 8 to 10 minutes, or until heated through.

Tip: Pork tenderloins are typically sold two to a pack. You can freeze the second tenderloin as is or double this recipe, stuff the second tenderloin, and wrap it tightly, uncooked, in foil and freeze for up to 3 months. Thaw completely before cooking as directed in the recipe.

Per Serving: Calories: 286; Total fat: 21g; Protein: 22g: Total carbs: 2g; Fiber: 1g; Net carbs: 1g

Macros: Fat: 66%; Protein: 31%; Carbs: 3%

Stovetop Chopped Pork Barbecue

Prep time: 10 minutes / **Cook time:** 40 minutes **Serves 6**

Many barbecue sauces are loaded with sugar and just don't work on a ketogenic diet. Here, I don't skip the flavor but use a vinegar-based sauce to keep carbs minimal. Using pork loin in place of a higher-fat shoulder not only helps the pork cook faster but also reduces the saturated fat in this dish. I add heart-healthy unsaturated fat with the olive oil to keep ketogenic ratios on point.

2 teaspoons paprika

2 teaspoons garlic powder

2 teaspoons onion powder

1½ teaspoons salt

½ to 1 teaspoon red pepper flakes

1½ pounds pork tenderloin or pork chops, cut into 2-inch pieces

½ cup extra-virgin olive oil

¼ cup apple cider vinegar or red wine vinegar

½ to 1 cup chicken or beef stock

1. In a medium bowl, whisk the paprika, garlic powder, onion powder, salt, and red pepper flakes to blend. Add the pork pieces and toss to coat well with the spices.

2. In a medium saucepan over medium-high heat, heat the oil. Add the pork and cook for about 5 minutes, stirring, to brown on all sides.

3. Slowly, to prevent splattering, pour in the vinegar and enough stock to cover the pork. Bring to a boil, reduce the heat to low, cover the pan, and simmer for 15 to 20 minutes, or until the pork is cooked through.

4. Using a slotted spoon, transfer the pork to a cutting board. Bring the liquid back to a boil, uncovered, and boil for 8 to 10 minutes, stirring occasionally, until the stock is reduced to just under 1 cup.

5. Finely dice the pork, return it to the hot liquid, and stir to combine well. Serve the pork warm with the cooking liquid.

6. Refrigerate leftover cooked pork in an airtight container for up to 4 days, or freeze for up to 3 months.

Tip: If you have a slow cooker, this pork turns even more tender when cooked over a longer period of time. Simply add all ingredients to the slow cooker, stir to combine, cover, and cook on low heat for 6 hours. Follow steps 4 and 5 to finish.

Per Serving: Calories: 312; Total fat: 22g; Protein: 26g; Total carbs: 1g; Fiber: 1g; Net carbs: 0g

Macros: Fat: 63%; Protein: 37%; Carbs: 0%

Eggplant Lasagna

Prep time: 15 minutes / **Cook time:** 50 minutes   **Serves 6**

Lasagna is not only the quintessential comfort food, but it also works great for prepping ahead and freezing or having fresh for a handful of meals. This dish is also perfect for entertaining or feeding a crowd if you want to double the recipe and use a larger dish. You could also make this vegetarian by omitting the beef.

4 tablespoons extra-virgin olive oil, divided

2 medium or 1 large eggplant, cut lengthwise into ¼-inch-thick slices

8 ounces ground beef

6 garlic cloves, minced, or 3 tablespoons jarred minced garlic

2 teaspoons Italian seasoning or dried oregano

1 teaspoon salt

¼ teaspoon freshly ground black pepper

1½ cups whole milk ricotta

2 large eggs, beaten

1½ cups shredded mozzarella cheese, divided

1 (24-ounce) jar no-sugar-added marinara sauce (such as Rao's)

1. Preheat the oven to 400°F. Line two baking sheets with parchment paper or aluminum foil and drizzle each with 1 tablespoon of oil, spreading it evenly.

2. Arrange the eggplant slices in a single layer on the prepared baking sheets.

3. Roast for 15 to 20 minutes until the eggplant is tender but not crispy. Remove from the oven and let cool to the touch.

4. Reduce the oven temperature to 375°F.

5. While the eggplant roasts, in a large skillet over medium-high heat, heat the remaining 2 tablespoons of oil. Add the ground beef and cook for 5 to 6 minutes, stirring, until browned and crumbly. Add the garlic, Italian seasoning, salt, and pepper and sauté for 1 to 2 minutes, or until fragrant. Remove from the heat.

6. In a small bowl, whisk the ricotta, eggs, and ½ cup of mozzarella to blend. Add the cheese mixture to the beef and stir to combine well.

7. Pour one-third of the marinara sauce (about 1 cup) into an 8×8-inch glass baking dish and spread it evenly over the bottom. Place 1 layer of roasted eggplant atop the sauce. Top the eggplant with one-third of the ricotta and beef mixture. Repeat with two more cycles of these layers: marinara, eggplant, and ricotta-beef. Top with the remaining 1 cup of mozzarella and cover the dish with aluminum foil.

8. Bake for 25 to 30 minutes, or until bubbly. Remove the foil and bake for 5 to 10 minutes, or until the cheese is slightly browned. Let cool for 5 minutes before slicing to serve.

9. Refrigerate leftover cooked lasagna in an airtight container for up to 5 days, or freeze for up to 3 months.

Per Serving: Calories: 508; Total fat: 36g; Protein: 25g; Total carbs: 23g; Fiber: 6g; Net carbs: 17g

Macros: Fat: 64%; Protein: 20%; Carbs: 16%

Chorizo and Peppers

Prep time: 5 minutes / **Cook time:** 20 minutes   **Serves 4**

Chorizo is a spicy pork sausage, native to Spain and often found in Latin American cuisine here in the States. Available in most U.S. grocery stores, you can find raw chorizo both in bulk and in casings. The deep spice flavor profile means very few added ingredients in this dish, keeping it simple yet bold and delicious. Substitute hot Italian pork sausage if you can't find chorizo.

1 pound raw ground pork chorizo, removed from its casing, if needed

2 tablespoons extra-virgin olive oil

½ medium onion, thinly sliced

1 red bell pepper, thinly sliced

1 yellow or orange bell pepper, thinly sliced

6 garlic cloves, thinly sliced or 3 tablespoons jarred minced garlic

1. Heat a large skillet over medium-high heat. Add the chorizo and cook for 6 to 8 minutes, breaking it into small crumbles, until it is crispy and most of the fat has been rendered. Using a slotted spoon, transfer the chorizo to a medium bowl, reserving the rendered fat in the skillet.

2. Add the oil to the fat in the skillet and heat for 1 minute. Add the onion and red and yellow bell peppers and sauté for 4 to 6 minutes until just tender. Add the garlic and return the cooked chorizo to the skillet. Reduce the heat to low, cover the skillet, and cook for 2 to 3 minutes until fragrant and the veggies are very tender. Serve warm.

3. Refrigerate leftover cooked chorizo and peppers in an airtight container for up to 4 days.

Tip: If you use chicken or turkey sausage, which is leaner, add 2 tablespoons olive oil when cooking it.

Per Serving: Calories: 423; Total fat: 35g; Protein: 17g; Total carbs: 11g; Fiber: 2g; Net carbs: 9g

Macros: Fat: 74%; Protein: 16%; Carbs: 10%

Pork Chops with Creamy Mushrooms

Prep time: 10 minutes / **Cook time:** 30 minutes **Serves 4**

Here's a great way to get your veggies. The rich sauce keeps the pork tender and works well for leftovers, also. Serve the sauce over chicken thighs or a hearty fish, such as swordfish or mahi-mahi, if you prefer.

4 (4-ounce) boneless pork chops

1½ teaspoons salt, divided

½ teaspoon black pepper, divided

2 tablespoons extra-virgin olive oil

2 tablespoons unsalted butter

½ small onion, thinly sliced

4 ounces sliced mushrooms

2 cups coarsely chopped baby spinach leaves, or ⅔ cup frozen spinach, thawed and drained

2 garlic cloves, minced, or 1 teaspoon garlic powder

¼ cup heavy (whipping) cream

¼ cup shredded Parmesan cheese

1. Season the pork chops with ½ teaspoon of salt and ¼ teaspoon of pepper.

2. In a large skillet over medium-high heat, heat the oil. Add the pork chops and sear for 3 to 4 minutes per side until browned. Remove from the skillet and keep warm.

3. Reduce the heat to medium and add the butter and onion. Sauté for 4 to 5 minutes until the onion is just tender. Add the mushrooms, remaining 1 teaspoon of salt, and the remaining ¼ teaspoon of pepper. Sauté for 4 to 5 minutes until just tender.

4. Add the spinach and garlic and sauté for 2 minutes. Whisk in the heavy cream and Parmesan and bring to a boil. Reduce the heat to low, return the pork chops to the skillet, cover the skillet, and cook for 5 to 6 minutes until the pork is cooked through and the sauce is thick and creamy. Serve the pork warm with the sauce spooned on top.

5. Refrigerate leftover cooked pork and sauce in an airtight container for up to 4 days.

Per Serving: Calories: 372; Total fat: 27g; Protein: 28g; Total carbs: 3g; Fiber: 1g; Net carbs: 2g

Macros: Fat: 65%; Protein: 30%; Carbs: 5%

Korean-Style Barbecue Beef Lettuce Cups

Prep time: 10 minutes, plus 20 minutes to marinate

Cook time: 10 minutes **Serves 4**

I love the sweet and spicy flavors of Korean barbecue, but most restaurant versions are loaded with sugar and typically served with a lot of rice. This keto-friendly adaptation uses lettuce leaves for serving and loads up on the flavor with fresh herbs and sliced avocado. For the best flavor, marinate the cut steak for at least 6 hours, or overnight.

1 pound beef skirt steak, thinly sliced

½ cup beef stock

½ cup sugar-free ketchup

¼ cup low-sodium soy sauce

¼ cup sesame oil

2 to 4 teaspoons granulated sugar-free sweetener (such as Swerve; optional)

1 tablespoon Sriracha or other hot sauce (optional)

4 garlic cloves, finely minced, or 2 tablespoons jarred minced garlic

2 teaspoons ground ginger

2 tablespoons extra-virgin olive oil

4 to 8 large Bibb or romaine lettuce leaves

½ to 1 cup fresh cilantro leaves

2 ripe avocados, peeled, pitted, and thinly sliced

1 lime, cut into wedges

1. In a large zip-top plastic bag, combine the steak, stock, ketchup, soy sauce, sesame oil, sweetener to taste (if using), Sriracha (if using), garlic, and ginger. Seal the bag and shake to mix well. Let marinate at room temperature for 20 minutes, or in the refrigerator for 6 hours to overnight.

2. In a medium skillet over high heat, heat the olive oil. Using a slotted spoon or tongs, remove the steak from the marinade and add it to the skillet. Reserve the marinade. Stir-fry the steak for 2 to 3 minutes until browned on all sides.

3. Pour the marinade into the skillet and bring it to a boil. Reduce the heat to low and simmer the mixture for 4 to 5 minutes, or until thickened and the beef is cooked through. Serve the beef warm in the lettuce leaves, garnished with cilantro and avocado. Serve the lime wedges on the side for squeezing.

4. Refrigerate leftover cooked beef in an airtight container for up to 4 days. Slice the avocado and chop the cilantro just before serving.

Per Serving: Calories: 489; Total fat: 38g; Protein: 27g; Total carbs: 13g; Fiber: 6g; Net carbs: 7g

Macros: Fat: 70%; Protein: 22%; Carbs: 8%

Mozzarella-Stuffed Sliders

Prep time: 10 minutes / **Cook time:** 15 minutes   Serves 6

Filled with gooey cheesy goodness, these little sliders are not your average burgers. The spinach adds a good dose of nutrition and fiber, but you can omit it and opt for a side salad or sautéed spinach instead. Serve these on the Everything but the Carb Bread (page 150), or, for a lighter meal, in lettuce wraps.

1 pound ground beef

⅔ cup frozen spinach, thawed and drained

¼ cup chopped olive oil–packed sun-dried tomatoes, with their oil

1 teaspoon garlic powder

½ teaspoon salt

¼ teaspoon freshly ground black pepper

3 (1-ounce) whole milk mozzarella cheese sticks, cut into 18 cubes

2 tablespoons extra-virgin olive oil

1. In a large bowl, combine the beef, spinach, sun-dried tomatoes and oil, garlic powder, salt, and pepper and mix well. Using your hands, form the meat mixture into 6 balls. Stick your thumb into the center of each ball to create a pocket and stuff 3 mozzarella cubes into each, then form the meat into a small patty shape around the cheese.

2. In a large skillet over medium-high heat, heat the oil. Add the burgers, cover the skillet, and cook for 5 to 6 minutes per side, or until the burgers are cooked to your desired doneness. Serve warm.

3. Refrigerate leftover sliders in an airtight container for up to 4 days, or wrap individually in aluminum foil and freeze for up to 3 months.

Tip: Leftover cooked burgers freeze nicely, but if you are only cooking for one or two, halve this recipe to make only 3 sliders to be used fresh for a couple of meals.

Per Serving: Calories: 301; Total fat: 22g; Protein: 24g; Total carbs: 3g; Fiber: 1g; Net carbs: 2g

Macros: Fat: 66%; Protein: 32%; Carbs: 2%

Sausage Ball Soup

Prep time: 10 minutes / **Cook time:** 30 minutes   Serves 6

Here is a fun spin on a classic party food to make a complete hearty meal on a cold night. Check the label on the sausage to ensure there is no sugar added. Use ground chicken or beef, if you prefer, but add 2 tablespoons of Italian seasoning for flavor.

1 pound bulk Italian sausage

1 cup finely shredded Cheddar cheese

¼ cup almond flour

1 teaspoon garlic powder

½ teaspoon salt

2 tablespoons extra-virgin olive oil

½ medium onion, thinly sliced

6 cups chicken stock

4 cups torn kale or baby spinach

1. In a large bowl, combine the sausage, cheese, almond flour, garlic powder, and salt and mix until well blended. Using your hands, form the mixture into roughly 16 (1-inch) balls and place them on a cutting board or large platter.

2. In a large stockpot or saucepan over medium-high heat, heat the oil. Add the onion and sauté for 4 to 5 minutes, or until just tender.

3. Very slowly, to prevent splatter, pour in the stock and bring to a boil over high heat. One by one, drop the sausage balls into the boiling liquid. Reduce the heat to low, cover the pot, and simmer for 15 minutes.

4. Add the kale to the pot, re-cover, and simmer for 4 to 5 minutes, or until the sausage is cooked through and the kale is tender. Serve the soup warm.

5. Refrigerate leftover soup in an airtight container for up to 4 days, or freeze for up to 3 months.

Tip: You can make the meatballs ahead and refrigerate them, uncooked, in an airtight container for up to 4 days. Add them to the pot in step 4.

Per Serving: Calories: 413; Total fat: 33g; Protein: 24g; Total carbs: 5g; Fiber: 1g; Net carbs: 4g

Macros: Fat: 72%; Protein: 23%; Carbs: 5%

Beef and Italian Sausage Ragù

Prep time: 5 minutes / **Cook time:** 30 minutes   **Serves 4**

Authentic Italian flavor that goes from stovetop to table in about 30 minutes, this is a great weekend supper go-to. The easy homemade marinara sauce can be made vegetarian by omitting the beef and pork and used in a variety of other recipes such as the Easiest Eggplant Parmesan (page 78) or the Chicken Margherita (page 104).

2 tablespoons extra-virgin olive oil

8 ounces ground beef

8 ounces Italian pork sausage, removed from its casing, if needed

½ small onion, diced

4 garlic cloves, minced

1 teaspoon salt

½ teaspoon black pepper

1 (28-ounce) can crushed tomatoes

1 tablespoon balsamic vinegar

2 teaspoons dried basil or Italian seasoning

8 cups spiralized zucchini noodles (zoodles)

1 to 2 teaspoons hot sauce (optional)

¼ cup grated Parmesan cheese (optional)

1. In a medium saucepan over medium-high heat, heat the oil. Add the ground beef and sausage and cook for 4 to 5 minutes, breaking up any clumps, until browned.

2. Add the onion and sauté for 4 to 5 minutes, or until the onion is just tender. Add the garlic, salt, and pepper and sauté for 2 minutes.

3. Pour in the crushed tomatoes and vinegar and stir in the basil to combine. Bring the mixture to a boil, reduce the heat to low, cover the pan, and simmer for 15 minutes.

4. Place the zucchini noodles in a large bowl and sprinkle with the hot sauce to taste (if using). Pour the ragù over the zoodles and toss to coat well. Divide evenly between 4 bowls. Garnish with grated Parmesan cheese (if using).

5. Refrigerate leftover sauce and zucchini noodles separately in airtight containers for up to 4 days. Add a dry paper towel to the zucchini noodles to absorb any moisture and prevent them from becoming mushy.

Per Serving: Calories: 483; Total fat: 30g; Protein: 28g; Total carbs: 25g; Fiber: 6g; Net carbs: 19g

Macros: Fat: 56%; Protein: 23%; Carbs: 21%

Steak and Blue Cheese Salad

Prep time: 10 minutes / **Cook time:** 15 minutes    **Serves 2**

This rich and flavorful salad is indulgent enough for a dinner party but simple enough for a weekday dinner or lunch. The recipe uses warm cooked steak, but you could make it even faster using leftover steak or rolled deli roast beef to cut down on prep time. The salad is fantastic with Tangy Blue Cheese Dressing, or use your favorite store-bought brand. Just be sure to pick one that has no sugar added.

1 (6-ounce) New York strip steak

½ teaspoon salt

¼ teaspoon freshly ground black pepper

2 tablespoons extra-virgin olive oil

4 cups baby arugula

2 tablespoons thinly slivered red onion

8 kalamata olives, pitted and halved

1 ounce crumbled blue cheese

4 tablespoons Tangy Blue Cheese Dressing (page 153), or store-bought blue cheese dressing

1. Season the steak with salt and pepper.

2. In a skillet over high heat, heat the oil. Add the steak and cook for 3 to 6 minutes per side, depending on the thickness of the cut and desired doneness. Remove from the skillet and let rest before slicing thinly.

3. While the steak cooks, divide the arugula between 2 bowls. Top each with half the red onion, olives, and blue cheese. Add the steak and drizzle each salad with 2 tablespoons of dressing. Serve warm.

Tip: This salad is best prepared fresh, but you can cook the steak ahead, prep all the ingredients, and assemble and dress the salad just before serving. Arugula is one of the most micronutrient-dense plant foods out there, and the peppery flavor is delicious in this salad. You can substitute any salad green for the arugula, if you prefer.

Per Serving: Calories: 524; Total fat: 44g; Protein: 24g; Total carbs: 7g; Fiber: 1g; Net carbs: 6g

Macros: Fat: 76%; Protein: 18%; Carbs: 6%

Keto Chili

Prep time: 10 minutes / **Cook time:** 35 minutes   **Serves 4**

All the flavor and comfort of traditional chili without all the carbs. This chili is even better served as leftovers after the spices have had time to develop. Serve garnished with a dollop of sour cream, chopped fresh cilantro, or sliced avocado. I like sliced black olives and scallions, too, for something different.

¼ cup extra-virgin olive oil

1 pound ground beef

½ medium onion, diced

2 medium poblano peppers or green bell peppers, diced

1 (4-ounce) can diced green chilies, undrained

4 garlic cloves, minced, or 2 tablespoons jarred minced garlic

1 teaspoon chili powder

1 teaspoon ground cumin

1 teaspoon dried oregano

1 teaspoon salt

¼ teaspoon freshly ground black pepper

4 cups beef or chicken stock

1. In a large stockpot or saucepan over medium-high heat, heat the oil. Add the ground beef and cook for 3 to 4 minutes, breaking up clumps, to brown. Add the onion and poblanos and sauté for 4 to 6 minutes, or until the beef is cooked through and the vegetables are just tender.

2. Add the green chilies and their juices, garlic, chili powder, cumin, oregano, salt, and pepper and sauté for 2 to 3 minutes, or until very fragrant.

3. Pour in the stock, bring to a boil, reduce the heat to low, cover the pot, and simmer for 15 to 20 minutes, or longer, until fragrant and thickened. Serve the chili warm.

4. Refrigerate leftover chili in an airtight container for up to 5 days, or freeze for up to 3 months.

Tip: For complete ease, this can be made in the slow cooker. Simply combine all ingredients in the cooker, cover, and cook on low heat for 4 to 6 hours.

Per Serving: Calories: 461; Total fat: 34g; Protein: 33g; Total carbs: 6g; Fiber: 1g; Net carbs: 5g

Macros: Fat: 66%; Protein: 29%; Carbs: 5%

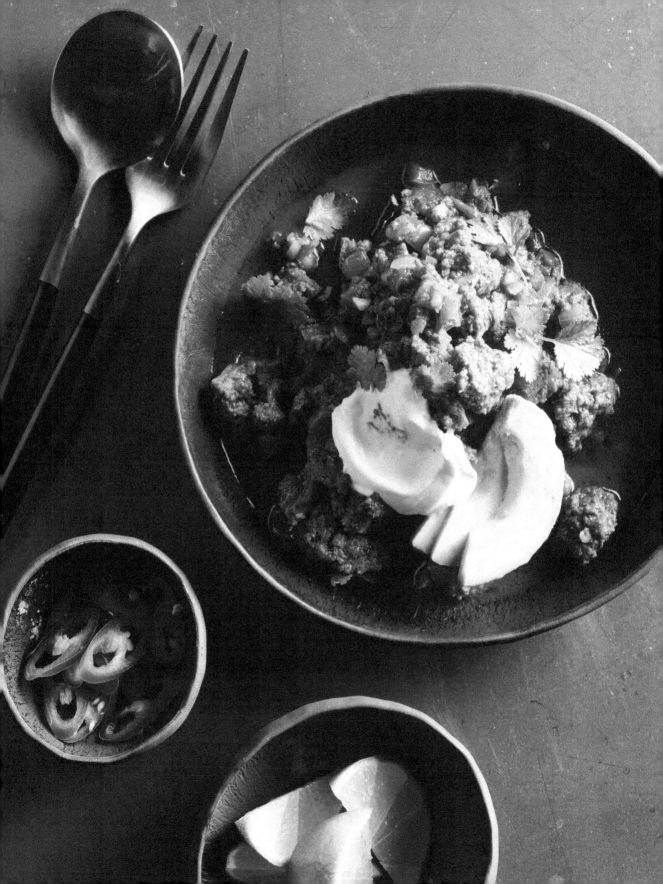

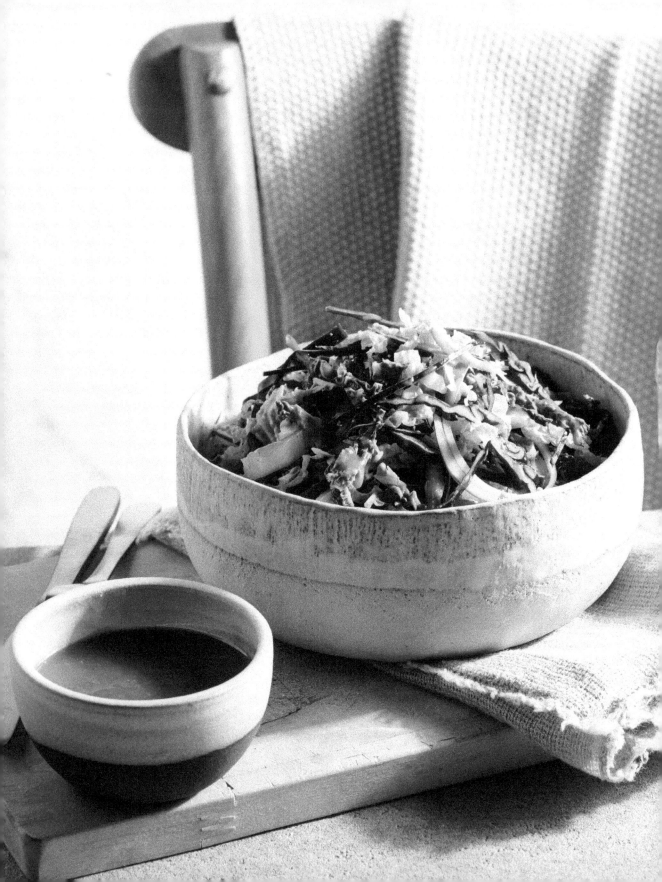

8

SNACKS AND SIDES

Chocolate-Almond Chia Pudding

Prep time: 5 minutes, plus 6 hours to chill    **Serves 4**

The heart-healthy and anti-inflammatory omega-3 fatty acids in chia seeds create a gel when dissolved in a liquid, forming the consistency of a pudding without any of the work. I love anything with chocolate and almonds to tackle that sweet tooth craving. Finish with a light sprinkle of sea salt for the salty-sweet winning taste combination.

1¾ cups unsweetened almond milk

¼ cup unsweetened almond butter

1 tablespoon unsweetened cocoa powder

1 to 2 teaspoons sugar-free sweetener (optional)

1 teaspoon almond or vanilla extract

½ cup chia seeds

1. In a medium bowl, whisk the almond milk, almond butter, cocoa powder, sweetener (if using), and almond extract until smooth and creamy.

2. Add the chia seeds and whisk until well combined.

3. Divide the mixture evenly between 4 ramekins or small jars. Cover and refrigerate for at least 6 hours. Serve cold.

4. Refrigerate leftover pudding in an airtight container for up to 1 week.

Tip: If your almond butter is cold and very thick, heat it in the microwave on high power for 15 to 20 seconds to melt it slightly so it is easier to blend with the liquid.

Per Serving: Calories: 238; Total fat: 18g; Protein: 8g; Total carbs: 15g; Fiber: 8g; Net carbs: 7g

Macros: Fat: 68%; Protein: 13%; Carbs: 19%

Baked Ricotta with Berries

Prep time: 5 minutes, plus 2 hours to chill (optional)

Cook time: 30 minutes   **Serves 2**

Much like one of my favorite Spanish desserts, the flan, this baked ricotta is light and airy but full of protein and healthy fats to keep it keto friendly. If you don't have ramekins or smaller ovenproof containers, double the recipe to make four servings and bake it in an 8 × 8-inch glass baking dish.

1 tablespoon unsalted butter

2 large eggs

2 teaspoons Swerve or other sugar-free sweetener of choice

1 teaspoon baking powder

1 teaspoon vanilla extract

½ teaspoon ground cinnamon

½ cup whole milk ricotta

¼ cup frozen mixed berries, thawed and chopped with their juices

1. Preheat the oven to 350°F. Coat the bottom and sides of 2 (1-cup) ovenproof ramekins or small glass containers with the butter.

2. In a medium bowl, whisk the eggs, sweetener, baking powder, vanilla, and cinnamon until smooth. Add the ricotta and berries and their juices and whisk until well blended. Divide the mixture evenly between the prepared baking dishes.

3. Bake for 25 to 30 minutes, or until set in the middle.

4. Baked ricotta can be eaten warm, or bring it to room temperature, cover, and refrigerate for at least 2 hours to serve chilled.

5. Refrigerate leftover ricotta in an airtight container for up to 4 days and serve chilled or warmed in the microwave.

Per Serving: Calories: 238; Total fat: 17g; Protein: 11g; Total carbs: 13g; Fiber: 1g; Net carbs: 8g

Macros: Fat: 64%; Protein: 18%; Carbs: 18%

Rosemary Nut and Olive Mix

Prep time: 10 minutes / **Cook time:** 15 minutes   **Makes 1¼ cups**

Nuts are a classic keto snack, but grabbing a handful of your go-to nuts gets old after a while. Here's a great way to mix it up with sweet and savory flavors in this quick and easy mix. These are fantastic served warm, fresh from the oven, or pop them in the microwave for 15 to 20 seconds for intense flavor.

1 cup assorted
  unsalted nuts (such
  as almonds, Brazil
  nuts, cashews,
  macadamia nuts,
  pecans, or walnuts)
¼ cup halved and
  pitted kalamata
  olives
1 tablespoon
  extra-virgin olive oil
1 tablespoon chopped
  fresh rosemary
  leaves, or 1 teaspoon
  dried
½ to 1 teaspoon red
  pepper flakes
½ teaspoon salt

1. Preheat the oven to 350°F. Line a baking sheet with aluminum foil.

2. In a medium bowl, combine the nuts, olives, oil, rosemary, red pepper flakes, and salt and toss to coat well. Spread the mixture in a single layer on the prepared baking sheet.

3. Roast for 10 to 12 minutes, or until the nuts are golden brown and the olives have dried out a bit. Let cool slightly before serving warm.

4. Refrigerate leftover nut mix in an airtight container for up to 3 weeks, or freeze for up to 3 months.

Tip: I love the simple flavors of rosemary and olive oil here, but switch it up by using other dried herbs. For a more Indian-inspired flavor, switch out the kalamata olives for green olives and use curry powder in place of the herbs.

Per Serving (2 tablespoons): Calories: 104; Total fat: 9g; Protein: 3g; Total carbs: 4g; Fiber: 1g; Net carbs: 3g

Macros: Fat: 78%; Protein: 12%; Carbs: 10%

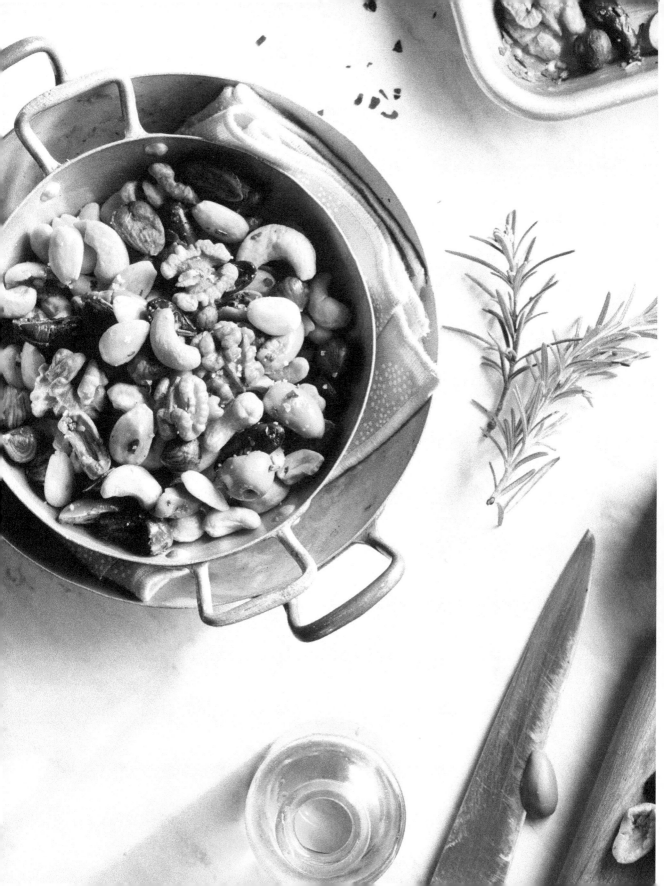

Sesame and Ginger Slaw

Prep time: 15 minutes   **Serves 4**

This slaw has an intense flavor and, combined with the crunch of the cabbage, it will soon be a favorite way to get in your veggies. Tahini is made from ground sesame seeds and is used in dips like hummus as well as to thicken sauces and dressings. It is typically found in either the international aisle of most grocery stores or with the other nut butters. If you can't find it, substitute unsweetened peanut butter or almond butter.

¼ cup tahini (sesame seed paste) or unsweetened peanut butter

2 tablespoons extra-virgin olive oil

2 tablespoons sesame oil

2 tablespoons soy sauce

2 tablespoons rice wine vinegar

1 tablespoon minced fresh ginger or ginger paste

2 cups thinly sliced red cabbage

2 cups thinly sliced napa or savoy cabbage

¼ small red onion, thinly sliced

1. In a large bowl, whisk the tahini, olive oil, sesame oil, soy sauce, vinegar, and ginger until smooth.

2. Add the red cabbage, napa cabbage, and red onion and toss to coat well. Serve immediately or let sit for up to 30 minutes at room temperature. Toss again before serving.

3. If making this ahead, refrigerate the dressing from step 1 and the cabbages and red onion in separate airtight containers for up to 1 week. Dress the slaw and toss just before serving.

Tip: You can use only one type of cabbage, if you prefer, but I love the variety for color and texture. Red cabbage is firmer and has more bite whereas the napa or savoy is more tender. To make this even easier, you can use 4 cups bagged coleslaw mix (no dressing).

Per Serving: Calories: 232; Total fat: 22g; Protein: 4g; Total carbs: 8g; Fiber: 3g; Net carbs: 5g

Macros: Fat: 85%; Protein: 7%; Carbs: 8%

Avocado Salad

Prep time: 10 minutes   Serves 4

This refreshing and easy-to-make salad is like a deconstructed bowl of guacamole—what could be better? Make this a complete meal by adding grilled chicken, shrimp, or steak, or serve alongside scrambled or fried eggs for a great brunch treat.

¼ cup extra-virgin olive oil

Juice of 1 lemon

1 teaspoon salt

½ teaspoon freshly ground black pepper

2 ripe avocados, peeled, pitted, and cut into 1-inch chunks

1 red bell pepper, cut into 1-inch chunks

¼ cup halved cherry tomatoes

¼ to ½ cup packed fresh cilantro leaves

¼ cup minced red onion

1 jalapeño pepper, seeded and chopped (optional)

1. In a small bowl, whisk the oil, lemon juice, salt, and pepper to combine. Set aside.

2. In a large bowl, combine the avocados, bell pepper, tomatoes, cilantro, red onion, and jalapeno (if using).

3. Drizzle the dressing over the salad and toss to coat.

4. Refrigerate leftovers in an airtight container for up to 2 days before the avocados get mushy and turn brown.

Tip: To prep this salad ahead, store the dressing separately, add the avocado when serving, and toss to coat and combine.

Per Serving: Calories: 251; Total fat: 24g; Protein: 2g; Total carbs: 10g; Fiber: 6g; Net carbs: 4g

Macros: Fat: 86%; Protein: 3%; Carbs: 11%

Italian Green Bean Salad

Prep time: 10 minutes, plus 30 minutes to chill (optional)

Cook time: 5 minutes   **Serves 4**

This easy side is delicious served warm or cold, depending on the season and your preference. I love this prepared ahead and served cold as a lunch salad or even as part of a summer potluck spread. It also makes a great side served warm alongside simple grilled meat, fish, or chicken.

4 tablespoons extra-virgin olive oil, divided

2 tablespoons balsamic vinegar

2 tablespoons minced red onion

2 teaspoons Italian seasoning or dried oregano, basil, or rosemary

1 garlic clove, finely minced, or 1 teaspoon garlic powder

1 teaspoon salt

½ teaspoon red pepper flakes or freshly ground black pepper

1 pound green beans, trimmed

½ cup thinly sliced fresh basil (optional)

1. In a large bowl, whisk 2 tablespoons of oil, the vinegar, red onion, Italian seasoning, garlic, salt, and red pepper flakes to combine. Set aside.

2. In a large skillet over medium-high heat, heat the remaining 2 tablespoons of oil. Add the green beans and sauté for 4 to 5 minutes, or until just tender. Transfer the beans to the bowl with the dressing. Add the fresh basil (if using) and toss well to coat. Serve the salad warm, or chill for at least 30 minutes to serve cold.

3. Refrigerate the salad in an airtight container for up to 4 days. Reheat in a skillet over medium-high heat for 2 to 3 minutes to serve warm, or serve cold.

Tip: This salad is also delicious made with broccoli, cauliflower, or asparagus prepared the same way. You can mix up the herbs, using fresh rosemary in place of the basil, or try thyme or tarragon for a French-inspired flair.

Per Serving: Calories: 167; Total fat: 14g; Protein: 2g; Total carbs: 11g; Fiber: 3g; Net carbs: 7g

Macros: Fat: 75%; Protein: 5%; Carbs: 20%

Smoked Salmon Roll-Ups

Prep time: 15 minutes   **Serves 4**

Smoked salmon and goat cheese go together like ham and Swiss, and these fun, easy-to-make little roll-ups make a great high-protein mid-afternoon snack. Double the serving size and pair it with mixed greens tossed with your favorite dressing for a complete meal.

4 ounces smoked salmon

2 ounces goat cheese

2 tablespoons extra-virgin olive oil

1 tablespoon minced fresh chives or scallions

1 teaspoon dried dill

1. On a cutting board, cut the thin slices of smoked salmon evenly into two equal rectangles. In each rectangle, the thin slices will be overlapping each other.

2. In a small bowl, stir together the goat cheese, oil, chives, and dill. Top each salmon rectangle with the goat cheese mixture and spread to coat evenly. Starting at the narrow end, roll the salmon to form a log. Halve each salmon roll to form 4 roll-ups.

3. To store, tightly wrap each roll-up individually in plastic wrap and refrigerate for up to 4 days. Serve chilled.

Tip: Substitute cream cheese or crème fraîche for the goat cheese if you are not a big fan of its flavor. Try deli ham or turkey in place of the salmon, if you prefer.

Per Serving: Calories: 145; Total fat: 12g; Protein: 8g; Total carbs: <1g; Fiber: <1g; Net carbs: <1g

Macros: Fat: 74%; Protein: 22%; Carbs: 4%

Roasted Brussels Sprouts with Feta and Balsamic Glaze

Prep time: 10 minutes / **Cook time:** 25 minutes **Serves 4**

The balsamic glaze adds a little touch of sweet to this savory side dish that will be sure to up your Brussels sprouts game. You can substitute crumbled goat cheese for the feta or omit it altogether for a vegan option.

1 pound Brussels
   sprouts, trimmed and
   halved, very large
   ones quartered
4 tablespoons
   extra-virgin olive oil,
   divided
1 teaspoon salt
¼ teaspoon freshly
   ground black pepper
¼ cup balsamic
   vinegar
2 ounces crumbled
   feta cheese

1. Preheat the oven to 400°F. Line a rimmed sheet pan with aluminum foil.

2. In a medium bowl, combine the Brussels sprouts, 2 tablespoons of oil, the salt, and the pepper and toss to coat. Spread the Brussels sprouts into a single layer on the prepared baking sheet. Do not rinse the mixing bowl.

3. Roast for 20 to 25 minutes, or until golden and crispy, turning the pan halfway through the cooking time.

4. While the Brussels sprouts roast, in a small skillet over medium-high heat, bring the vinegar to a boil. Reduce the heat to low and simmer, stirring frequently, for 10 to 15 minutes until thickened and reduced by half. Remove from the heat.

5. Return the roasted Brussels sprouts to the bowl and drizzle with the remaining 2 tablespoons of oil and the reduced vinegar. Add the feta and toss to coat. Serve warm.

6. Refrigerate leftovers in an airtight container for up to 4 days. Reheat in the microwave to serve warm.

Tip: You can find prepared balsamic glaze next to the vinegars and oils in most grocery stores, but be sure there is no sugar added. The commercial glaze will be thicker and higher in sugar, so use only 1 tablespoon of the glaze in step 5.

Per Serving: Calories: 220; Total fat: 17g; Protein: 6g; Total carbs: 14g; Fiber: 4g; Net carbs: 10g

Macros: Fat: 70%; Protein: 11%; Carbs: 19%

Guacamole Deviled Eggs

Prep time: 10 minutes   **Serves 4**

Guacamole meets deviled eggs for a match made in snack heaven. Filled with heart-healthy omega-3 fats and added fiber from the avocado, this rich and filling high-protein snack is sure to nip any craving in the bud. Made ahead, these are a great on-the-go breakfast for busy weekend mornings.

4 store-bought peeled hard-boiled eggs

½ medium ripe avocado, peeled and pitted

1 tablespoon extra-virgin olive or avocado oil

2 tablespoons minced red onion

2 tablespoons chopped fresh cilantro (optional)

1 garlic clove, finely minced, or 1 teaspoon garlic powder

1 teaspoon salt

¼ teaspoon freshly ground black pepper

1. Halve the hard-boiled eggs lengthwise and scoop the yolks into a medium bowl. Place the 8 egg white halves, cut-side up, on a plate or in a storage container.

2. To the yolks, add the avocado and oil and mash well with a fork until smooth and creamy. Stir in the red onion, cilantro (if using), garlic, salt, and pepper well to combine. Spoon the filling into each egg white half.

3. Serve immediately, or cover and refrigerate for up to 48 hours. If you want to prep this ahead, refrigerate the egg whites and filling in separate airtight containers for up to 4 days and fill just before serving. To delay the avocado from browning, store the guacamole with plastic wrap pressed tightly over it, touching the surface of the mixture, to prevent oxygen from reaching it.

Tip: Using store-bought hard-boiled eggs means this recipe comes together in a flash, but you can boil your own eggs, chill, and peel them before making this recipe. Refrigerate unpeeled hard-boiled eggs for up to 1 week.

Per Serving (2 filled egg halves): Calories: 140; Total fat: 11g; Protein: 7g; Total carbs: 3g; Fiber: 1g; Net carbs: 2g

Macros: Fat: 71%; Protein: 20%; Carbs: 9%

Dilled Cucumber Salad

Prep time: 10 minutes, plus time to chill (optional)   **Serves 4**

So light and refreshing, this is a great way to use plentiful garden cucumbers in summer. This version of cucumber salad deviates from the Southern staple a bit with the addition of olives, but I love the briny flavor mixed with the dill, creamy mayo, and crunchy cucumber. I like using avocado oil mayonnaise here for its added anti-inflammatory health benefit, not to mention great taste, but use your favorite mayonnaise as you prefer.

¼ cup mayonnaise

1 tablespoon red wine vinegar

1 teaspoon dried dill, or 1 tablespoon chopped fresh dill

½ teaspoon salt

¼ teaspoon freshly ground black pepper

20 pitted kalamata olives, halved (about ½ cup)

1 large English (seedless) cucumber, cut into half-moon shapes

1. In a large bowl, whisk the mayonnaise, vinegar, dill, salt, and pepper until smooth and creamy.

2. Add the olives and the cucumber half-moons and stir to combine well. Serve chilled or at room temperature.

3. Refrigerate leftover salad in an airtight container for up to 3 days.

> **Tip:** You can peel the cucumber, if you prefer, but leftovers hold up better with the peel left on. The peel also provides an extra crunchy texture.

Per Serving: Calories: 170; Total fat: 16g; Protein: 1g; Total carbs: 5g; Fiber: 1g; Net carbs: 4g

Macros: Fat: 85%; Protein: 2%; Carbs: 13%

Southwestern Cottage Cheese Salad

Prep time: 5 minutes, plus time to chill   **Serves 1**

I know not everyone loves cottage cheese, but the mixture of tastes and textures in this simple high-protein and healthy-fat combo may just convert even the strongest skeptic. I like this served as a savory breakfast or as a light lunch. Mix in arugula or chopped romaine lettuce to bulk it up.

½ cup full-fat cottage cheese

1 teaspoon taco seasoning or chili powder

½ avocado, peeled, pitted, and diced

2 tablespoons chopped fresh cilantro

2 tablespoons roasted pumpkin seeds

Hot sauce, for seasoning (optional)

1. In a small bowl, stir together the cottage cheese and taco seasoning until well combined.

2. Add the avocado, cilantro, and pumpkin seeds and gently stir to incorporate well without mashing the avocado. Season to taste with hot sauce (if using). Serve cold.

3. Refrigerate the salad in an airtight container for up to 4 hours if making ahead for later in the day, but I do not recommend prepping it in advance for later in the week.

Tip: Trader Joe's sells an "everything but the elote" seasoning that is fantastic here, or use your favorite seasoning blend, such as curry powder or everything bagel seasoning.

Per Serving: Calories: 312; Total fat: 22g; Protein: 18g; Total carbs: 14g; Fiber: 6g; Net carbs: 8g

Macros: Fat: 63%; Protein: 23%; Carbs: 14%

Energy Balls

Prep time: 15 minutes, plus 30 minutes to chill   **Makes 6 balls**

These are a go-to in my household to replace store-bought granola or snack bars. With real ingredients and just enough sweetness to stave off a sugar craving, I recommend doubling the recipe and storing half in the freezer to have on hand. You can use any unsweetened nut butter that you prefer—peanut, macadamia, cashew, etc.

½ cup unsweetened almond butter, at room temperature

½ cup almond flour

1 tablespoon sugar-free sweetener (optional)

2 tablespoons unsweetened coconut flakes

1 tablespoon chia seeds

½ teaspoon ground cinnamon

1. In a medium bowl, stir together the almond butter, almond flour, and sweetener (if using) until well combined. If your almond butter is very thick or cold, microwave it on high power for 15 to 20 seconds to make it smoother and easier to blend.

2. Add the coconut flakes, chia seeds, and cinnamon and mix to incorporate well. Using your hands, form the mixture into 6 (1-inch) balls.

3. Place the balls in a single layer in a storage container and refrigerate for at least 30 minutes before serving to harden. Once they harden, you can transfer them to a zip-top plastic bag to make storage easier.

4. Refrigerate the energy balls in an airtight container for up to 2 weeks, or freeze for up to 3 months.

> **Tip:** To make these a higher-protein post-workout snack, replace the almond flour with your favorite protein powder (no sugar added) to increase the protein by about 5 grams per serving.

Per Serving (1 ball): Calories: 203; Total fat: 18g; Protein: 7g; Total carbs: 7g; Fiber: 4g; Net carbs: 3g

Macros: Fat: 80%; Protein: 14%; Carbs: 6%

Caprese Cheese Spread

Prep time: 10 minutes   **Serves 4**

Creamy and satiating, pimento cheese, which is traditionally made with shredded Cheddar and Duke's mayonnaise mixed with jarred pimientos, is an easy keto-friendly snack or light meal. This is my spin on the Southern classic using fresh mozzarella, pesto, and sun-dried tomatoes. Fill celery sticks or romaine lettuce leaves with this gooey, savory treat, or make a grilled cheese sandwich using Everything but the Carb Bread (page 150) or spread on Rosemary and Olive Oil Crackers (page 146) for a more filling meal.

¼ cup jarred pesto or Versatile Pesto (page 149)

1 tablespoon mayonnaise

4 ounces fresh mozzarella, shredded

2 tablespoons chopped olive oil–packed sun-dried tomatoes, with their oil

1. In a medium bowl, whisk the pesto and mayonnaise until smooth and creamy.

2. Stir in the mozzarella and sun-dried tomatoes and oil until well combined.

3. Refrigerate the cheese spread in an airtight container for up to 1 week.

Tip: This is my ideal version of pimento cheese using my personal favorite flavors, but get creative and make this your own by using your favorite shredded cheese and flavored sauce. Try Swiss cheese, equal parts garlic aïoli, and stone-ground mustard with chopped pickles for more of a Reuben spin, or go with tradition using shredded Cheddar, mayonnaise, and jarred pimientos or roasted red peppers.

Per Serving: Calories: 227; Total fat: 21g; Protein: 9g; Total carbs: 5g; Fiber: 1g; Net carbs: 4g

Macros: Fat: 83%; Protein: 16%; Carbs: 1%

Cream of Broccoli Soup

Prep time: 10 minutes / **Cook time:** 30 minutes   **Serves 4**

Even my clients who struggle with getting in their veggies love this as a side option for any main protein. Creamy and rich, it also makes a comforting lunch or light dinner on a cold day. You could substitute cauliflower or asparagus for the broccoli, if you prefer.

¼ cup extra-virgin olive oil

½ medium onion, slivered

2 cups broccoli florets, broken into small pieces

4 garlic cloves, coarsely chopped, or 2 tablespoons jarred minced garlic

1 teaspoon dried thyme

1 teaspoon salt

½ teaspoon freshly ground black pepper

4 cups chicken or vegetable stock

½ cup heavy (whipping) cream

½ cup shredded Cheddar cheese (optional)

1. In a medium saucepan over medium heat, heat the oil. Add the onion and sauté for 4 to 6 minutes until just tender.

2. Add the broccoli and garlic and sauté for 3 to 4 minutes, or until the broccoli is lightly browned and the garlic is fragrant.

3. Stir in the thyme, salt, and pepper. Pour in the stock and heavy cream and bring the mixture to a boil. Reduce the heat to low, cover the pan, and simmer for 12 to 15 minutes, or until the broccoli is very tender.

4. Remove from the heat and stir in the cheese (if using). Using an immersion blender, puree the soup until smooth and creamy. Or, cool slightly and transfer to a standard blender. Serve warm.

5. Refrigerate leftover soup in an airtight container for up to 1 week. Reheat in the microwave or on the stovetop before serving.

Per Serving: Calories: 257; Total fat: 24g; Protein: 6g; Total carbs: 5g; Fiber: 2g; Net carbs: 3g

Macros: Fat: 84%; Protein: 9%; Carbs: 7%

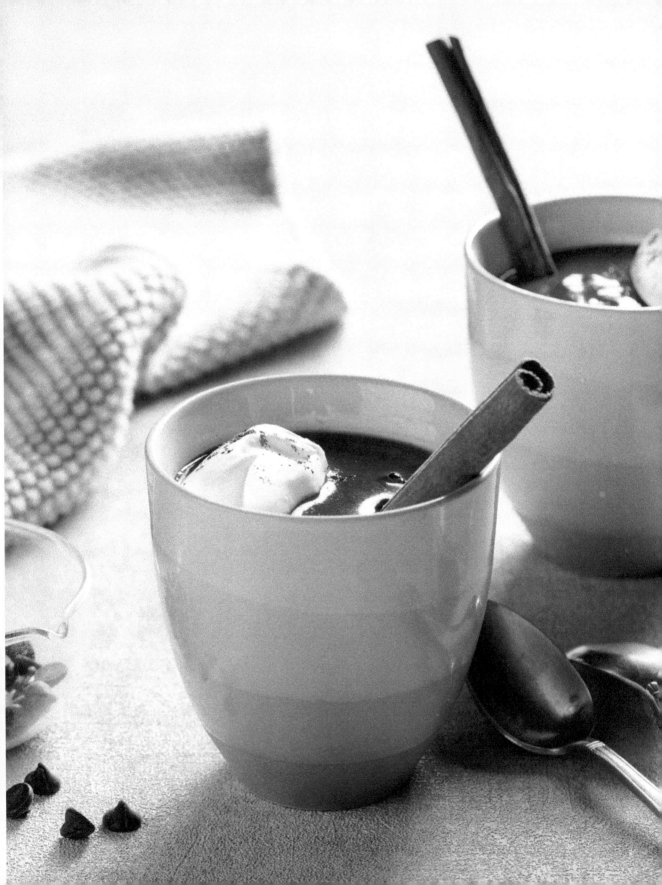

9

STAPLES

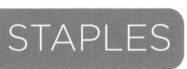

Rosemary and Olive Oil Crackers

Prep time: 20 minutes / **Cook time:** 15 minutes **Serves 6**

Sometimes you just need a crunch, and these easy-to-make crackers will satisfy that need. Great on their own, they also make a great dipping vessel for the Caprese Cheese Spread (page 142) or Curried Tuna Salad (page 94) for a light lunch or heavy snack.

1 cup almond flour

1 teaspoon dried rosemary or Italian seasoning

1 teaspoon onion powder

½ teaspoon garlic powder

½ teaspoon salt

¼ teaspoon baking soda

1 large egg, at room temperature

2 tablespoons extra-virgin olive oil

Per Serving (3 or 4 crackers): Calories: 163; Total fat: 15g; Protein: 5g; Total carbs: 4g; Fiber: 2g; Net carbs: 2g

Macros: Fat: 83%; Protein: 12%; Carbs: 5%

1. Preheat the oven to 350°F. Line a baking sheet with parchment paper.

2. In a medium bowl, whisk the almond flour, rosemary, onion powder, garlic powder, salt, and baking soda until well combined.

3. In a small bowl, whisk the egg and oil to blend. Add the wet ingredients to the dry ingredients and stir until well combined. Using your hands, form the dough into a ball.

4. Place one layer of parchment paper on a work surface and place the dough on top. Cover with a second layer of parchment paper and, using a rolling pin, roll the dough to ⅛-inch thickness, aiming for a rectangular shape. Remove the top layer of parchment and cut the dough into 2-inch-square crackers. Transfer the crackers to the prepared baking sheet on the parchment.

5. Bake for 10 to 15 minutes, or until crispy and slightly golden. Let cool slightly before serving.

6. Store leftover crackers in an airtight container at room temperature for up to 4 days, or in the refrigerator for up to 1 week. Bring to room temperature before serving.

Keto Granola Bites

Prep time: 5 minutes / **Cook time:** 20 minutes

Makes 18 (1-inch) squares

Full of all the crunch and flavor of traditional granola without all the sugar and carbs, these little bites of pure snack heaven are also rich in omega-3 fatty acids, helping reduce inflammation and improve heart health.

2 tablespoons unsalted butter, melted

2 to 4 teaspoons sugar-free sweetener (optional)

1 teaspoon vanilla extract

½ cup slivered almonds

½ cup roasted pumpkin seeds

¼ cup ground flaxseed

¼ cup chia seeds

1 large egg white, beaten

Per Serving (3 squares): Calories: 214; Total fat: 18g; Protein: 8g; Total carbs: 8g; Fiber: 5g; Net carbs: 3g

....

Macros: Fat: 76%; Protein: 15%; Carbs: 9%

1. Preheat the oven to 350°F. Line a baking sheet with parchment paper.

2. In a small bowl, whisk the butter, sweetener (if using), and vanilla until smooth. Set aside.

3. In a medium bowl, combine the almonds, pumpkin seeds, flaxseed, and chia seeds. Stir in the egg white. Add the butter mixture and stir until well combined. Spread the mixture into a thin layer, about ½ inch thick, on the prepared baking sheet.

4. Bake for 18 to 20 minutes, or until golden, being careful not to burn the granola. Remove from the oven and let cool for 5 minutes.

5. Cut the baked granola into 1-inch squares. Store in an airtight container or zip-top plastic bag at room temperature for up to 1 week, or freeze for up to 3 months.

Tip: You can turn these bites into more of a crumbled granola to use atop yogurt. Spread the granola into a thinner ¼-inch layer before baking and reduce the baking time to 12 to 15 minutes. Crumble once cooled and store in a sealed container for up to 1 week.

Mexican-Inspired Drinking Chocolate

Prep time: 5 minutes / **Cook time:** 2 minutes  Serves 1

This is your go-to for when your inner chocoholic starts screaming. Small, yet comforting and rich, this drink is just enough to tame the craving without compromising your goals. I love the strong cinnamon spice flavor of Mexican chocolate and find that when cutting back on sugar, loading up on other flavors helps keep your taste buds satisfied. Omit the cinnamon and cayenne, if you prefer.

1 ounce sugar-free chocolate chips (such as Lily's)

¼ cup heavy (whipping) cream

½ teaspoon vanilla extract

⅛ teaspoon ground cinnamon

Pinch cayenne pepper (optional)

1. In a small microwave-safe mug or bowl, combine the chocolate, heavy cream, and vanilla. Microwave on high power for 1 minute. Stir and microwave for another 30 to 60 seconds, or until the chocolate is melted. Stir or whisk until the mixture is very smooth.

2. Whisk in the cinnamon and cayenne (if using) and serve warm.

Tip: In place of the sugar-free chips, which can be pricey, use 1 ounce unsweetened baking chocolate and 1 to 2 teaspoons sugar-free sweetener to taste.

Per Serving: Calories: 321; Total fat: 30g; Protein: 4g; Total carbs: 18g; Fiber: 8g; Net carbs: 6g

Macros: Fat: 84%; Protein: 5%; Carbs: 11%

Versatile Pesto

Prep time: 5 minutes   **Makes about 1 cup**

So many of my clients struggle with creative ways to get all the healthy fats into their meals to keep ratios in check yet feel satiated with meals. My answer is sauces, sauces, and more sauces! Pesto, or a simple herb, garlic, and olive oil combination, is so easy to make and so full of flavor it can really jazz up any meal—from simple grilled meats, fish, or chicken to scrambled eggs, roasted veggies, or even as a dressing for salads. Traditional pesto is made with basil and pine nuts, but any herb and nut combination will do for similar texture and intense flavor.

4 cups packed fresh herbs
1 cup nuts, chopped
½ cup extra-virgin olive oil
2 small garlic cloves, minced
1 teaspoon salt

In a blender, combine the herbs, nuts, oil, garlic, and salt and blend until very finely chopped and smooth. Transfer the mixture to an airtight container, preferably glass, and refrigerate, covered, for up to 2 weeks.

Tip: This recipe works with any combination of herbs and nuts, so get creative and use what you have on hand. Some of my favorite combinations are parsley and pecan; sage, arugula, and walnut; cilantro and cashew; mint and almond; and, of course, basil and pine nut or almond.

Per Serving (2 tablespoons): Calories: 232; Total fat: 24g; Protein: 3g; Total carbs: 4g; Fiber: 2g; Net carbs: 2g

Macros: Fat: 93%; Protein: 5%; Carbs: 2%

Everything but the Carb Bread

Prep time: 5 minutes / **Cook time:** 2 minutes   Makes 2 bread rounds

Although they may follow ketogenic ratios, extra calories and non-net carbs from keto-friendly commercial breads can really add up. This simple recipe uses real food ingredients for an easy at-home solution for when you just want a sandwich or a piece of toast or are in the mood for a warm roll with your dinner meal without sacrificing weight-loss goals.

Nonstick cooking spray
1 large egg
3 tablespoons almond flour
1 tablespoon extra-virgin olive oil
1 teaspoon everything bagel seasoning, or ⅛ teaspoon salt
½ teaspoon baking powder

1. Coat 2 (6-ounce) microwave-safe ramekins or mugs with cooking spray.

2. In a small bowl, whisk the egg, almond flour, oil, everything bagel seasoning, and baking powder until well combined. Divide the mixture evenly between the prepared containers. One at a time, microwave each on high power for 90 seconds. Let cool for 2 minutes.

3. Slide a knife around the inside edges of each ramekin and flip to remove the bread. Using a serrated knife, halve the bread horizontally if you want to use it to make a sandwich or thin toast, or enjoy it whole as a roll.

4. Wrap the bread tightly in aluminum foil or plastic wrap and refrigerate for up to 4 days. Bring to room temperature, or microwave on high power for 10 to 15 seconds before serving.

Tip: If you don't have a microwave, bake the bread in a 375°F oven for 8 to 10 minutes until a toothpick inserted into the center comes out clean.

Per Serving (1 bread round): Calories: 169; Total fat: 15g; Protein: 5g; Total carbs: 4g; Fiber: 1g; Net carbs: 3g

Macros: Fat: 80%; Protein: 12%; Carbs: 8%

Molly's Special Sauce

Prep time: 5 minutes   Makes 1 cup

Another simple way to add flavorful healthy fats to meals without getting bored, this sauce is great with grilled fish, meats, or vegetables as well as spread onto lettuce or low-carb wraps along with your favorite lunch meat or salad for a stellar "sandwich" option. If you like spicy sauces, add a dash of hot sauce or Sriracha for a bit of heat.

½ cup mayonnaise

½ cup no-sugar-added ketchup

1 kosher pickle, minced

1 teaspoon garlic powder

1 teaspoon onion powder

1 teaspoon salt

¼ teaspoon smoked paprika

In a small bowl, whisk the mayonnaise, ketchup, pickle, garlic powder, onion powder, salt, and paprika until smooth and creamy. Serve immediately, or refrigerate in an airtight container for up to 2 weeks.

Tip: You can make this your special sauce by adding your favorite spice blends. Some of my favorite variations are curry, chipotle or chili powder, and dried tarragon.

Per Serving (2 tablespoons): Calories: 107; Total fat: 10g; Protein: <1g; Total carbs: 2g; Fiber: <1g; Net carbs: 2g

Macros: Fat: 84%; Protein: <1%; Carbs: 16%

Coconut and Lime Sauce with Basil

Prep time: 5 minutes / **Cook time:** 15 minutes   Makes 2 cups

Thick, creamy, and full of Thai-inspired flavors, this sauce is great for dipping or topping grilled fish or chicken, or thin it with a bit of stock or water and use as a simmer sauce to cook chunks of a protein over low heat or in a slow cooker to infuse amazing flavor and body into a meal.

1 (13.5-ounce) can
   full-fat coconut milk
Grated zest of 2 limes
4 garlic cloves, minced,
   or 2 tablespoons
   jarred minced garlic
Juice of 2 limes
¼ cup packed thinly
   sliced fresh basil
   leaves
2 tablespoons fish
   sauce or soy sauce

1. In a small saucepan over medium-high heat, whisk the coconut milk, lime zest, and garlic to blend. Bring to a boil, whisking frequently. Reduce the heat to low and simmer for 10 to 15 minutes, or until thickened.

2. Remove the sauce from the heat and whisk in the lime juice, basil, and fish sauce. Serve warm.

3. Refrigerate leftovers in an airtight container for up to 1 week.

> **Tip:** The fresh basil adds great flavor, but you can substitute mint or cilantro, or omit the herbs entirely for a different taste profile.

Per Serving (½ cup): Calories: 176; Total fat: 17g; Protein: 2g; Total carbs: 8g; Fiber: 1g; Net carbs: 7g

Macros: Fat: 87%; Protein: 5%; Carbs: 8%

Tangy Blue Cheese Dressing

Prep time: 10 minutes   **Makes about 1 cup**

This thick, creamy dressing, loaded with chunks of blue cheese, makes a wonderful dipping sauce for raw veggies or spicy chicken wings, and is perfect with the Steak and Blue Cheese Salad (page 123). This version is easy to make and so much richer in flavor, you'll never go back to store-bought blue cheese dressing.

3 ounces crumbled blue cheese

¼ cup buttermilk, plus more as needed

¼ cup full-fat sour cream

¼ cup mayonnaise

1 teaspoon garlic powder

1 teaspoon onion powder

½ teaspoon salt

¼ teaspoon freshly ground black pepper

1. Place the blue cheese in a medium bowl or glass jar and mash with a fork into very small crumbles. Add the buttermilk and whisk with the fork until well combined.

2. Add the sour cream, mayonnaise, garlic powder, onion powder, salt, and pepper and whisk until well combined. Whisk in additional buttermilk to thin the dressing to your desired consistency.

3. Refrigerate the dressing in an airtight container for up to 2 weeks.

Tip: This makes a thick dressing that holds up as a great dipping sauce. If you prefer a thinner dressing, increase the buttermilk to ⅓ cup or more.

Per Serving (2 tablespoons): Calories: 106; Total fat: 10g; Protein: 3g; Total carbs: 2g; Fiber: <1g; Net carbs: 2g

Macros: Fat: 85%; Protein: 11%; Carbs: 4%

Creamy Caesar Dressing

Prep time: 5 minutes   **Makes 1½ cups**

Hands down, this is my go-to salad dressing and the most frequently asked-for recipe when I host a dinner party. It's so easy to make in bulk and I suggest keeping a jarful in the refrigerator to dress up your greens.

1 cup mayonnaise

Juice of 1 lemon (2 to 3 tablespoons)

1 tablespoon Dijon mustard

1 tablespoon Worcestershire sauce

1 teaspoon garlic powder

1 teaspoon onion powder

1 to 2 teaspoons anchovy paste (optional)

½ teaspoon salt

½ teaspoon freshly ground black pepper

In a small bowl or glass container with a lid, combine the mayonnaise, lemon juice, mustard, Worcestershire sauce, garlic powder, onion powder, anchovy paste (if using), salt, and pepper. Whisk until smooth and creamy. Serve immediately, or tightly cover and keep refrigerated for up to 2 weeks. Shake or whisk well before serving.

Tip: If you've never tried anchovy paste, you are missing out. It gives this dressing its unique umami flavor, but if you prefer, omit it.

Per Serving (2 tablespoons): Calories: 130; Total fat: 14g; Protein: <1g; Total carbs: 1g; Fiber: <1g; Net carbs: 1g

Macros: Fat: 97%; Protein: <1%; Carbs: 3%

Cilantro Lime Crema

Prep time: 5 minutes   **Makes about 1½ cups**

This is the stuff that makes fajita and taco bowls come to life. So simple yet full of zesty flavor, this sauce not only goes with Latin-inspired dishes, but also enhances any grilled meat, fish, or chicken and is fantastic with a couple scrambled eggs with avocado.

1 cup full-fat sour cream

½ cup packed fresh cilantro leaves

¼ cup avocado oil or olive oil

1 garlic clove, smashed

Juice of 1 lime (about 1 tablespoon)

1 teaspoon salt

¼ teaspoon freshly ground black pepper

In a blender, combine the sour cream, cilantro, oil, garlic, lime juice, salt, and pepper and blend until smooth and creamy. Serve immediately, or refrigerate in an airtight container for up to 1 week.

Tip: If you're not a fan of cilantro, use another herb, such as parsley or mint, for an equally creamy and refreshingly versatile sauce.

Per Serving (¼ cup): Calories: 159; Total fat: 17g; Protein: 1g; Total carbs: 3g; Fiber: <1g; Net carbs: 3g

Macros: Fat: 96%; Protein: 2%; Carbs: 2%

Alfredo Sauce

Prep time: 5 minutes / **Cook time:** 15 minutes   **Makes 1½ cups**

In my opinion, Alfredo sauce just makes everything taste better! This is a very rich and calorie-dense sauce, so it can help jazz up a leaner protein such as chicken breast or shrimp. Simply sauté the protein in a bit of olive oil until browned, add the sauce, cover, and simmer until the sauce is warmed and the protein is cooked through. Serve with zucchini noodles or over a bed of sautéed greens for a simple weeknight supper.

2 tablespoons
  unsalted butter
3 garlic cloves, minced
8 ounces full-fat
  cream cheese
½ cup heavy
  (whipping) cream
½ cup shredded
  Parmesan cheese
1 teaspoon salt
½ teaspoon freshly
  ground black pepper

1. In a medium saucepan over medium-low heat, melt the butter. Add the garlic and sauté for 2 to 3 minutes, or until very fragrant.

2. Add the cream cheese and heavy cream and cook, whisking, for 4 to 5 minutes, or until the cream cheese melts and mixture is smooth and creamy.

3. Whisk in the Parmesan, salt, and pepper and cook for 4 to 5 minutes, stirring frequently, until the cheese melts and the sauce is very smooth.

4. Remove from the heat and serve immediately, or cool completely, place in an airtight container, and refrigerate for up to 1 week. Reheat the sauce in the microwave or on the stovetop over low heat before serving.

Tip: If Alfredo makes everything better, pesto makes Alfredo even better. Substitute ¼ cup jarred or prepared Versatile Pesto (page 149) for ¼ cup of the heavy cream for a real treat.

Per Serving (¼ cup): Calories: 264; Total fat: 26g; Protein: 6g; Total carbs: 4g; Fiber: <1g; Net carbs: 4g

Macros: Fat: 89%; Protein: 9%; Carbs: 2%

Tzatziki

Prep time: 5 minutes   **Makes about 1½ cups**

A staple in Greek cuisine, tzatziki is a creamy, refreshing sauce served alongside grilled chicken, meats, and vegetables, and I love to use it as a thick dressing on salads. Try it with the Curry Roasted Chicken Thighs (page 105) or Nutty Riced Cauliflower (page 80).

½ cucumber, peeled, seeded, and coarsely chopped

1 cup full-fat plain Greek yogurt

¼ cup extra-virgin olive oil

2 tablespoons fresh dill, or 2 teaspoons dried dill

1 garlic clove, smashed

1 teaspoon salt

½ teaspoon freshly ground black pepper

In a blender, combine the cucumber, yogurt, oil, dill, garlic, salt, and pepper and blend until smooth and creamy. Serve immediately, or refrigerate in an airtight container for up to 1 week.

Tip: You can buy English, or seedless, cucumbers, usually wrapped in plastic in the produce department of most grocery stores. To seed a standard cucumber, peel it using a vegetable peeler, and quarter it vertically. Stand up each cucumber quarter and, using a knife, slice down to remove the seeds.

Per Serving (¼ cup): Calories: 117; Total fat: 11g; Protein: 4g; Total carbs: 2g; Fiber: <1g; Net carbs: 2g

Macros: Fat: 85%; Protein: 14%; Carbs: 1%

EXERCISES

CARDIO

Whether you are currently following a regular physical activity routine or just getting started incorporating more movement into your days, the three routines that follow provide some structure and guidance around timing and intensity to help you make this a reality. The activity you choose for each routine is up to what you like and what is available to you. For example, if you have a stationary or pedal bike, you may choose cycling. If you have a treadmill or prefer walking outdoors, walking or jogging may be your preference. For those with access to a pool or who enjoy the water, swimming may be your activity of choice.

I suggest aiming for at least 4 or 5 days a week of cardio activity for a minimum of 10 to 15 minutes each day, building up to 30 to 45 minutes per session. Consistency is always the goal so aim for shorter duration with more regularity to get you into a routine.

Routine Option #1: Beginner

1. Begin with a light 3- to 5-minute stretch to warm your muscles and prevent injury.

2. Transition to 10 to 30 minutes of low- to moderate-intensity movement (biking, jogging, light swimming, walking, etc.). You want to get your blood pumping, but you should be able to pass the "talk test," which is to carry on a conversation without being short of breath.

3. Finish with a light 3- to 5-minute stretch to cool down and prevent injury.

4. You may want to start with 10 minutes and gradually increase the duration by 5-minute increments every week until you feel you are ready for the next level of intensity.

Routine Option #2: Moderate

1. Begin with a light 3- to 5-minute stretch to warm your muscles and prevent injury.

2. Transition to 20 to 45 minutes of moderate-intensity movement (biking, light jogging, rowing, swimming, walking, etc.), with intervals of higher intensity as follows with an example of walking/jogging:

   - Five minutes of moderate-intensity walking, being able to pass the "talk test"

   - Thirty seconds to 1 minute of higher-intensity jogging or running to elevate your heart rate outside of the "talk test" zone

   - Repeat cycle, ending with a 1- to 2-minute lower-intensity walk to bring your heart rate back to baseline.

3. Finish with a light 3- to 5-minute stretch to cool down and prevent injury.

Routine Option #3: Advanced

1. Begin with a light 3- to 5-minute stretch to warm your muscles and prevent injury.

2. Transition to 20 to 45 minutes of higher-intensity activity (biking, jogging, rowing, swimming, etc.), with an elevated heart rate outside of the "talk test" zone. You can achieve this by increasing elevation on a treadmill or seeking out a hillier running coarse, increasing resistance on a bike or rowing machine, or including interval training in a pool.

3. Switch to 5 to 10 minutes of a low- to moderate-intensity "cooldown" (bike, light jog, swim, walk, etc.).

4. Finish with a light 3- to 5-minute stretch to prevent injury.

STRENGTH TRAINING

The following strength routines are designed to use a combination of body weight and free weights. The first beginner routine uses simple body weight resistance activities whereas the second two include the use of additional free weights. If you do not have free weights at home, use soup cans or modify the exercises using resistance bands.

Routine Option #1: Beginner

1. Begin with a light 3- to 5-minute stretch to warm your muscles and prevent injury.

2. Do 10 jumping jacks.

3. Switch to arm and leg extensions, holding for 30 seconds per side.

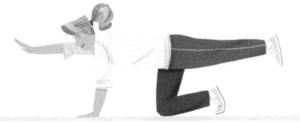

4. Do 10 sit-ups.

5. Do 10 squats.

6. Do 5 modified push-ups, either on your knees or with hands against a wall.

Routine Option #2: Moderate

1. Begin with a light 3- to 5-minute stretch to warm your muscles and prevent injury.

2. Do 15 jumping jacks.

3. Do 15 sit-ups.

4. Do 15 glute raises.

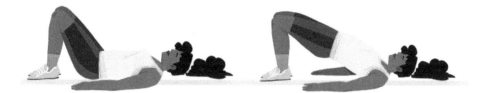

5. Do 15 double bicep curls with weight.

6. Do 10 modified push-ups, either on your knees or with hands against a wall.

Routine Option #3: Advanced

1. Begin with a light 3- to 5-minute stretch to warm your muscles and prevent injury.

2. Do 20 jumping jacks.

3. Do 20 abdominals with weights.

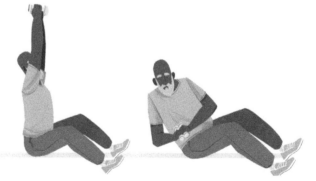

4. Do 20 (10 for each side) bicep curl/leg extensions with weight.

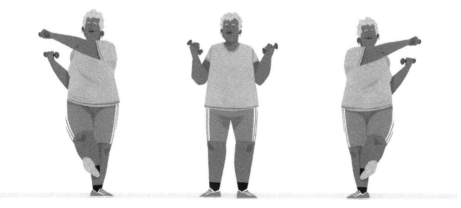

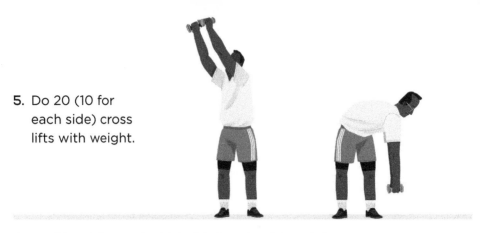

5. Do 20 (10 for each side) cross lifts with weight.

6. Do 20 (10 for each side) side bends with weight.

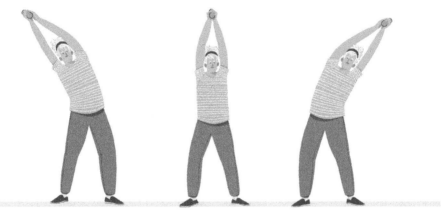

7. Do 20 modified push-ups, either on your knees or against a wall.

STRETCHING

The following is a 3- to 5-minute stretching routine you can use on rest days, or before and after cardio and strength training activities listed in the previous sections.

1. Hold a side bend for a count of 30 for each side (1 minute total).

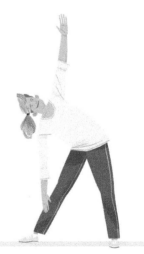

2. Perform a seated stretch to touch toes, bending knees if needed, for a count of 15. Rest and repeat.

3. Do knee lifts to elbows—10 on each side.

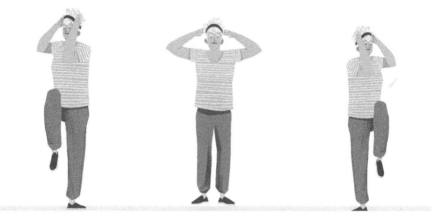

4. Arm across chest for a count of 30 for each arm.

5. Reach up to the sky. Hold for a count of 5. Then, reach down to your toes. Hold for a count of 5. Repeat 3 times.

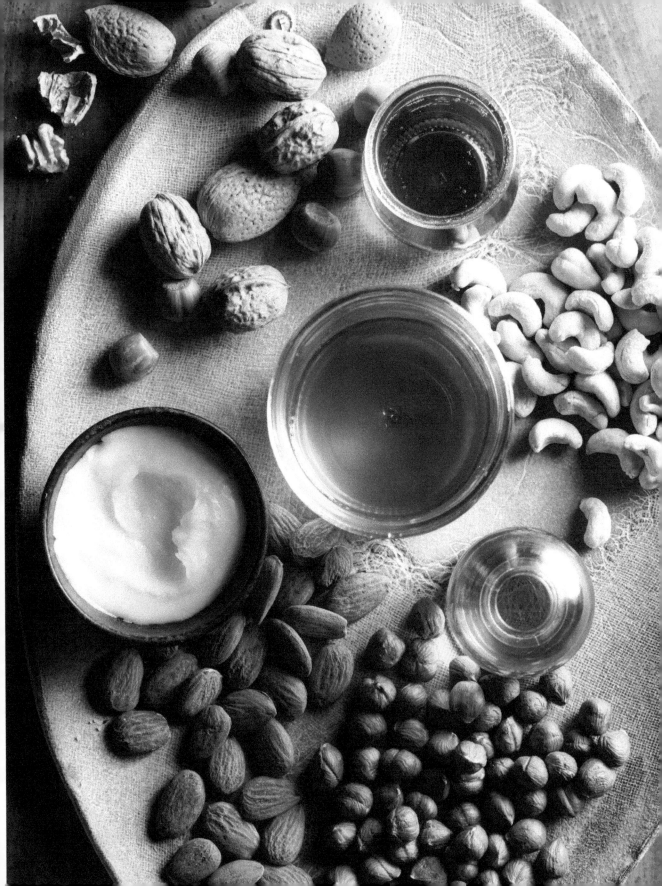

MEASUREMENT CONVERSIONS

VOLUME EQUIVALENTS	U.S. STANDARD	U.S. STANDARD (OUNCES)	METRIC (APPROXIMATE)
LIQUID	2 tablespoons	1 fl. oz.	30 mL
	¼ cup	2 fl. oz.	60 mL
	½ cup	4 fl. oz.	120 mL
	1 cup	8 fl. oz.	240 mL
	1½ cups	12 fl. oz.	355 mL
	2 cups or 1 pint	16 fl. oz.	475 mL
	4 cups or 1 quart	32 fl. oz.	1 L
	1 gallon	128 fl. oz.	4 L
DRY	⅛ teaspoon	–	0.5 mL
	¼ teaspoon	–	1 mL
	½ teaspoon	–	2 mL
	¾ teaspoon	–	4 mL
	1 teaspoon	–	5 mL
	1 tablespoon	–	15 mL
	¼ cup	–	59 mL
	⅓ cup	–	79 mL
	½ cup	–	118 mL
	⅔ cup	–	156 mL
	¾ cup	–	177 mL
	1 cup	–	235 mL
	2 cups or 1 pint	–	475 mL
	3 cups	–	700 mL
	4 cups or 1 quart	–	1 L
	½ gallon	–	2 L
	1 gallon	–	4 L

OVEN TEMPERATURES

FAHRENHEIT	CELSIUS (APPROXIMATE)
250°F	120°C
300°F	150°C
325°F	165°C
350°F	180°C
375°F	190°C
400°F	200°C
425°F	220°C
450°F	230°C

WEIGHT EQUIVALENTS

U.S. STANDARD	METRIC (APPROXIMATE)
½ ounce	15 g
1 ounce	30 g
2 ounces	60 g
4 ounces	115 g
8 ounces	225 g
12 ounces	340 g
16 ounces or 1 pound	455 g

REFERENCES

Campos, H., J. J. Genest Jr., E. Blijlevens, J. R. McNamara, J. L. Jenner, J. M. Ordovas, P. W. Wilson, et al. "Low Density Lipoprotein Particle Size and Coronary Artery Disease." *Arteriosclerosis and Thrombosis: A Journal of Vascular Biology* 12 (1992): 187–195. doi.org/10.1161/01.ATV.12.2.187.

Chianese, R., R. Coccurello, A. Viggiano, M. Scafuro, M. Fiore, G. Coppola, F. F. Operto, et al. "Impact of Dietary Fats on Brain Functions." *Current Neuropharmacology* 16, no. 7 (2018): 1059–1085. doi.org/10.2174/1570159X15666171017102547.

Chung, H. Y., D. H. Kim, E. K. Lee, K. W. Chung, et al. "Redefining Chronic Inflammation in Aging and Age-Related Diseases: Proposal of the Senoinflammation Concept." *Aging and Disease* 10, no. 2 (2019): 367–382. dx.doi.org/10.14336/AD.2018.0324.

D'Abbondanza, M., S. Ministrini, G. Pucci, E. Nulli Migliola, E. E. Martorelli, V. Gandolfo, D. Siepi, et al. "Very Low–Carbohydrate Ketogenic Diet for the Treatment of Severe Obesity and Associated Non-Alcoholic Fatty Liver Disease: The Role of Sex Differences." *Nutrients* 12, no. 9 (2020): 2748. doi.org/10.3390/nu12092748.

Fontana, Luigi, Samuel Klein, John O. Holloszy, and Bhartur N. Premachandra. "Effect of Long-Term Calorie Restriction with Adequate Protein and Micronutrients on Thyroid Hormones." *Journal of Clinical Endocrinology & Metabolism* 91, no. 8 (August 1, 2006): 3232–3235. doi.org/10.1210/jc.2006-0328.

Gasior, M., M. A. Rogawski, and A. L. Hartman. "Neuroprotective and Disease-Modifying Effects of the Ketogenic Diet." *Behavioural Pharmacology* 17 nos. 5–6 (2006): 431–439. doi.org/10.1097/00008877-200609000-00009.

Harvard Health Publishing. "Lessons from 'The Biggest Loser.'" Accessed January 17, 2022. health.harvard.edu/diet-and-weight-loss/lessons-from-the-biggest-loser.

Kosinski, C., and F. R. Jornayvaz. "Effects of Ketogenic Diets on Cardiovascular Risk Factors: Evidence from Animal and Human Studies." *Nutrients* 9, no. 5 (2017): 517. doi.org/10.3390/nu9050517.

Livestrong.com. "Does Eating a Low-Carb Diet Affect Bowel Movements?" Accessed October 29, 2020. livestrong.com/article/509998-do-low-carbs-affect-bowel-movements.

Mavropoulos, John C., William S. Yancy, Juanita Hepburn, and Eric C. Westman. "The Effects of a Low-Carbohydrate, Ketogenic Diet on the Polycystic Ovary Syndrome: A Pilot Study." *Nutrition & Metabolism* 2 (2005): 35. doi:10.1186/1743-7075-2-35.

Mobbs, C. V., J. Mastaitis, F. Isoda, and M. Poplawski. "Treatment of Diabetes and Diabetic Complications with a Ketogenic Diet." *Journal of Child Neurology* 28, no. 8 (2013): 1009–1014. doi.org/10.1177/0883073813487596.

Rhoads, Timothy W., and Rozalyn M. Anderson. "Taking the Long View on Metabolism." *Science* 373, no. 6556 (2021): 738–739. doi/10.1126/science.abl4537.

Vidali, S., S. Aminzadeh, B. Lambert, T. Rutherford, W. Sperl, B. Kofler, and R. G. Feichtinger. "Mitochondria: The Ketogenic Diet—A Metabolism-Based Therapy." *International Journal of Biochemistry & Cell Biology* 63 (2015): 55–59. doi.org/10.1016/j.biocel.2015.01.022.

Włodarek, D. "Role of Ketogenic Diets in Neurodegenerative Diseases (Alzheimer's Disease and Parkinson's Disease)." *Nutrients* 11, no. 1 (2019): 169. doi.org/10.3390/nu11010169.

Wood, Richard J., Jeff S. Volek, Yanzhu Liu, Neil S. Shachter, John H. Contois, and Maria Luz Fernandez. "Carbohydrate Restriction Alters Lipoprotein Metabolism by Modifying VLDL, LDL, and HDL Subfraction Distribution and Size in Overweight Men." *Journal of Nutrition* 136, no. 2 (2006): 384–389. doi.org/10.1093/jn/136.2.384.

INDEX

ABOUT THE AUTHOR

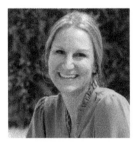 **Molly Devine** is a registered dietitian who specializes in digestive health, healthy weight management, and chronic disease prevention through integrative and functional nutrition. She is an advocate for sustainable lifestyle change through nutrition intervention and founder of MSD Nutrition Consulting, a nutrition counseling and individualized meal-planning service focusing on customized whole foods–based diets for disease prevention and management. She utilizes insurance-based telehealth to work with clients across the country on their health and nutrition goals. Find out more at msdnutrition.com, or email her at hello@msdnutrition.com.

Devine is the author of the *Anti-Inflammatory Keto Cookbook, Essential Ketogenic Mediterranean Diet Cookbook, Keto After 50, Keto Prediabetes Diet Plan, Keto Fitness Cookbook, The Complete Keto Meal Plan Cookbook, 30-Minute Vegiterranean Cookbook,* and *The Natural Candida Cleanse: A Healthy Treatment Guide to Improve Your Microbiome,* and is a contributor to nutrition-based online media such as *Shape Magazine, Insider, Greatist, HuffPost, Brides Magazine,* and ABC11 *Eyewitness News.*

Devine received her Bachelor of Science in Nutrition Sciences from North Carolina Central University and completed her Dietetic Internship through Meredith College. She also holds a Bachelor of Science in Languages and Linguistics from Georgetown University. She lives in Durham, North Carolina, with her family.

Printed in the USA
CPSIA information can be obtained
at www.ICGtesting.com
CBHW042352200124
3539CB00002B/5